Emmet Densmore

# The Natural Food of Man

A Brief Statement of the Principal Arguments Against the use of Bread,

Cereals, Pulses, etc.

Emmet Densmore

**The Natural Food of Man**
*A Brief Statement of the Principal Arguments Against the use of Bread, Cereals, Pulses, etc.*

ISBN/EAN: 9783744646031

Printed in Europe, USA, Canada, Australia, Japan

Cover: Foto ©Andreas Hilbeck / pixelio.de

More available books at **www.hansebooks.com**

# THE NATURAL FOOD OF MAN:

*A brief statement of the principal arguments against the use of Bread, Cereals, Pulses, and all other Starch Foods.*

BY

## EMMET DENSMORE, M.D.

"Our first duty is to become healthy."—*Heine.*

LONDON:

PEWTRESS AND CO., 28, Little Queen Street, Holborn, W.C.

NEW YORK: 319, W. 45th Street.

———

Price in Cloth, 2/- ; Paper Boards, 1/-.

# PREFACE.

---

The following pages, except the Introduction, are a re-publication of essays somewhat hurriedly written, partly in New York and partly in this country, while engrossed with professional and business cares. If there appears needless repetitions, especially in the Introduction, I ask attention to the following lines from Professor Max Muller :—" Repeat the same things over and over again, undismayed by indifference, ridicule, contempt, and all other weapons which the lazy mind knows so well how to employ against those who venture to disturb their peace by suggesting unwelcome truths."

If the central thought—that bread is the staff of death rather than life—seems preposterous and absurd, I can only urge that many of the accepted teachings of science to-day would not have seemed less so a hundred years ago.

After all, no amount of argumentation can settle this question. A few months' trial—with many, a few weeks—will show such results that arguments become quite unnecessary ; and all, I think, must agree that if the main teaching of this little book is based on truth, it is scarcely possible to exaggerate its importance.

In addition to the matter of health, of prime concern to every human being, I ask attention to another leading claim that friends of the non-starch diet make in its behalf. Nearly all Temperance reformers unite in affirming that the drink crave is brought on and kept alive by any habit or pursuit that tends to

weaken the nervous system. This may be tobacco, stimulating
food and drink, over-strain in physical or mental work, or undue
solicitude or excitement, from whatever cause. *Anything that
diminishes nerve nutrition is a prime cause of drunkenness.* That which
the inebriate, when trying to reform, most needs is an abundance
of wholesome nourishment, digested and assimilated with least
strain upon the nervous system. I have long been a student of
the drink problem, and am confident that the system of diet
herein advocated is invaluable to the Temperance workers ; that
anyone who can be persuaded to adopt this course of life is sure
to overcome all desire for intoxicating drinks already existing, and
that it will prevent the almost world-wide craving for narcotics
and stimulants of all kinds.

London, August, 1890.

# INTRODUCTION.

" 'Tis life, not death, for which we pant ;
'Tis life whereof our nerves are scant :
More life and fuller that we want."
— *Tennyson.*

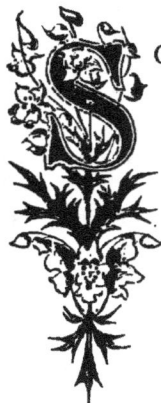

SOME ten years ago, while engaged in a study of the best foods to be used in the reduction of obesity, my mind became directed toward a matter of much greater import ; I became convinced that the great bulk of all modern diseases is directly caused by errors in diet ; and also that the illness of myself and friends, which I had been accustomed to attribute to heredity, or, more vaguely, to unfavourable conditions of climate, and business cares, and overwork, was and is the result of transgressions easily avoidable ; that, to the enlightened mind, to be ill is as reprehensible as to be drunk. Moreover, I perceived that man's natural longevity has been greatly abridged ; that the three-score years and ten, which I had been accustomed to regard as a well-rounded and mature life, is full fifty years short of our natural term ; and that a death at seventy is as untimely and premature as at forty, differing only in degree. And, while I did not omit from the account a consideration of the importance of fresh air, exercise, bathing, moderation in work, clothing, etc., I became convinced that more than ninety per cent. of all diseases result from unsuitable food and errors in eating and drinking.

Looking about me, I observed that men and women of forty and fifty years of age bear almost no resemblance to the appearance they presented at the age of twenty. Most women are beautiful at twenty, and generally (when regarded with a trained eye) hideous at fifty. Men have fared no better than women. The "human form divine" has lost its rightful contour, and approached in resemblance the jelly-fish. I early saw that obesity, or corpulency, is a kind of tumour—less unsightly than those tumours located in any given portion of the frame, but a tumour, all the same. Those who are not obese have not escaped ; marked faces, stiffened joints, and contorted bodies, are seen upon every hand ; and the emaciated are not less revolting than the obese. Old age, which should be a crown of glory, a perfected picture of a well-spent life, is too often a hideous deformity, a wreck of imbecility more or less idiotic.

My good brethren in the Temperance movement can see, with me, the pitiful wreck of the confirmed drunkard ; but do not see that it is only a part and parcel of the universal ruin. I dedicated my life to a study of those laws the transgr ession of which has made of the human race a collec-tive invalid, and to a propaganda of that knowledge best calculated to restore man to his first and best inheritance—Health !

I became a Vegetarian ; adopted that diet which see med at the time best calculated to overcome disease ; from a periodically pronounced inval'd, I became relatively robust, and restored to health. I was ena bled to obey that unique injunction, " Physician, heal thyself ! " and, in conjunction with Mrs. Densmore, was enabled to do for patients what we had done for ourselves. Our success, as compared with the results of other methods of practic:—Allopathic, Homœopathic, and Eclectic alike—was wonderful ; but it did not satisfy us. We supposed that brown bread is the " staff of life "—the sheet-anchor of hygienic cure. We believed that all seasonings and all animal foods are forbidden by the laws of health. As a crutch to lean upon, a bridge from the diet of civilisation to the ideal diet, we re-commended an exclusive use of brown bread and milk. The only medi-cine used was a mild herb-tea, to stimulate the excretory functions. Our success was signal ; it seemed only a question of inducing the confirmed invalid to obey our simple directions—a very difficult task—to bring about a rapid improvement, and sometimes a complete restoration of the patient.

We then began, with the best intentions, to wo rk serious evil to our patients. We felt ambitious to give them the whole gospel ; we supposed that brown bread and fruit contain every needed element ; we regarded milk and eggs as an unclean food, and only temporarily allowable, and re-commended the substitution of pulse foods as the best way of obtaining needed nitrogen. One dear lady came to us a mountain of flesh, and a confirmed invalid. At first we put her on an exclusive diet of beef and hot water, until she was reduced to a normal weight. This required some months ; and, by the time the obesity was gone, much of her infirmity had gone with it. We then put her on a diet of brown bread and milk, with water—no other food nor drink. Her recovery continued, until she was esteemed by herself and neighbours a marvellous cure. We then substi-tuted peas and beans for the milk. She had considerable trouble ; but it was not at first pronounced, and we confidently hoped, each week, that she would be better next. Finally, she was taken down with a severe inflamination of the stomach and bowels. From this attack she never fully re covered ; and we had many similar cases.

On the other hand, many patients, against our advice, adhered to a strict diet of bread and milk, with fruits, and continued the good health this riegimen had brought them. Some obese patients, whom we reduced on a meat diet and non-starch vegetables, and who had been greatly improved n health, were persuaded by us to adopt a bread, fruit, and pulse diet, and surprised us by developing serious troubles, for which we could find no satisfactory explanation. Others, again, declined our proffer of Vegetarian ism, adhering to a diet of meat and non-starch foods. These continued the good health they had gained. These patients did not refuse f od from any idea that it is injurious, but because they easily took on too much weight. We were greatly puzzled.

Last September (1889) I suggested to Mrs. Densmore the hypothesis that starch foods are unnatural and injurious ; that the reason why our obese patients, confined to an exclusively meat and non-starch d et, invari- ably gained in health as they lost in weight, is not so much—as we had supposed—that their infirmities had been caused by their obesity and were overcome by the reduction of the obesity, but that all starch food is favourable to disease, that our patients' infirmities were caused by starch (usually bread and potatoes), and the removal of the cause overcame the disease. The puzzle of a meat diet—stigmatised by us as excremental and unwholesome—working wonderful cures, was solved : the benefit did not result from flesh-food *per se*, but from the absence of cereals and other starch foods. This view was at once strengthened and confirmed by the plain fact that the successful treatment, the world around, for obesity and diabetes, is the elimination of all starch foods from the dietary ; and the probability dawned upon me that cereals, the universal food, are the primal source of universal disease.

Looking further, I perceived, what now seems strange had not before been dwelt upon by physiologists, that the process of digestion confirms and reaffirms the position that all starch foods are injurious, and furnishes the why and wherefore, in the fact that starch foods are not adapted to stomach digestion, and can only be made assimilable by protracted and difficult digestion in the intestines. I saw that this discovery—that starch foods, especially cereals, are an universal and unsuspected source of world- wide disease—is of the gravest possible importance to mankind. I was in America ; my mind at once adverted to my Vegetarian friends in England, and I felt that I must call their attention to this new view.

I wrote a letter, which was published in the *Vegetarian* last November, stating that Mrs. Densmore and myself had noticed remarkable cures result from taking all starch food from patients, and confining them to a meat diet. Incidentally, I pointed out that these cures had occurred in a practice of the reduction of obesity ; but asked that prominent Vegetarian physicians and hygienists would explain, from a Vegetarian standpoint, why it is that a meat diet quite uniformly works great benefits. My friends replied through the *Vegetarian*, utterly ignoring my question, with a deluge of free advice as to the best way to reduce obesity. I replied to these efforts, pointing out the fact that obesity and its reduction was not the subject of discussion ; and appealed to them to devote their powers to an answer to my question. Then came a deluge of a different sort. Dr. Allinson, a prominent Vegetarian physician, likened my efforts to " orange-peel thrown upon the pavement, from which the wise steer clear, and by which the unwary are thrown upon their backs." * Mr. Wallace, also a prominent Vegetarian physician, charged me with " playing cards with both God and the devil." Mr. Hills, the distinguished President of the London Vegetarian Society, and the head and front of the movement, accused me of " playing fast-and-loose with principles." What these unseemly out-bursts had to do with a scientific discussion, is more than I have been able to discern. One writer, only last month, under a nom-de-plume, but commonly identified as the distinguished author posing as the well-known and especial friend of animals, designated—by implication—my poor self an ass, and likened myself to a cannibal, and my writings to cannibalism. One Irish gentleman (?), whose name is unknown to fame—perhaps with an inherited shillalah—early in the fray, said that I am no Vegetarian, that I am " an enemy, stabbing Vegetarianism under the guise of friendship"; and then, after my most earnest protestations, and after months for consideration, returns to the charge, and, in a recent issue of the *Vegetarian*, says that I am " laughing up my sleeve at the gullibility of Vegetarians " ; while, as if to give piquancy to this true Hibernianism, he commenced his letter, from which the above quotation is taken, with a plea for Christian charity !

By frequent letters and rejoinders, which the Editor of the *Vegetarian* has been good enough to publish, I pointed out to my friends that my own shortcomings are not the subject of discussion ; that epithets and assertions are not argument ; and, by dint of that perseverance which is said to wear away stone, I succeeded in June in getting, from Mr. Hills and

---

* It is but fair to state that, since the above was i type, and months after Dr. Allinson made the above statement in the *Vegetarian*, he wrote another letter to that paper, from which I quote the following : " To Dr. Densmore I owe an apology ; instead of saying his ideas are ' mere speculation, and unfounded on fact or experience,' I should have said that ' his ideas are unfounded on experience, and unconfirmed by experiment,' and ask him to show me results which will justify his assertions. And instead of saying his articles were like orange-peel, that would throw unwary people down, I should have said they must be taken with a grain of salt."

others, some consideration of the question I had asked the previous November.

In the *Weekly Times and Echo*, June 21st, Dr. Allinson says :

" I do not believe in the 'nut and fruit' theory, as it is not founded on fact, not supported by proof, nor borne out by experience. In cases of disease it would be very injurious."

Dr. Allinson is in error; the "nut and fruit" theory is founded on a most important and indisputable scientific fact, namely : nuts and fruits contain, as demonstrated by chemical analysis, all the elements of nutrition needed for the support of man, and some varieties contain those elements in about the needed proportions. "Not supported by proof, nor borne out by experience"! Many of the negroes in the West Indies live on a diet consisting only of a measured amount of bananas. At the moment of writing I am not able to lay my hand on the authority for this statement ; but I have often seen it stated in accounts given by travellers, and I think the statement will not be challenged. I consider this as "proof," and that it is "borne out by experience," that the banana is not only a food adequate to keep up the heat of the body, and support the vital functions, but also— since these negroes were slaves, and performed regular tasks of manual labour—that the banana is a food furnishing ample support to the muscular system. A man may be careless about food for himself or his family ; but, when his cattle or his slaves are in question, his pocket is involved ; and man is a very conservative being, not at all given to fads or nonsense where his bank balance is in danger.

But let us look further. The promoters of the " nut and fruit theory " have never recommended an entire reliance upon those nuts and fruits which are usually obtainable in England, especially at a reasonable expense ; on the contrary, we have laid great stress and urgency in pointing out that it is best to supplement a diet of fruit and nuts with as much milk and eggs as may be found necessary or advisable. Here we are on safe ground ; we are "supported by proof, borne out by experience," that milk alone is an entirely adequate diet. Moreover, let us bear in mind that the "fruit and nut theory," just now agitating the minds of Vegetarians in England, is not that fruit and nuts, as here obtainable, are an adequate diet for man ; the fruit and nut theory asserts that cereals, pulses, and vegetables, are an unnatural and disease-inducing food for man ; the proof adduced, in support of this position, is the plain fact that patients afflicted with the diseases of diabetes and corpulency are always benefited and frequently cured by excluding starch foods from the dietary. The correctness of this assertion (the unwholesomeness of cereals) is further confirmed and "supported by the proof," and "borne out by the experience," of those patients of Dr. Salisbury, in America and England, who, exclusive of diabetes and obesity, have been greatly benefited, in all varieties of diseases to which man is subject, by an exclusive diet of beef and hot water, which is one way of excluding cereals, pulses, and vegetables from the dietary. This view is further confirmed by the " fact " that the foods which the promoters of the " nut and fruit theory " recommend, are adapted to stomach digestion, and are readily and easily digested and assimilated ; whereas the cereals are largely composed of those substances which are not adapted to stomach digestion, and which must be subjected to a protracted and difficult digestion in the intestines.

This view is, again, further confirmed by those scientific facts which Dr. De Lacy Evans has so ably set forth, that the cereals and pulses are loaded with those earthy matters which are shown to be the cause of the ossification and decrepitude of old age ; whereas nuts and fruit and eggs— truth being always homogeneous—are shown to be just those foods least apt to induce the ossification and the consequent decrepitude of old age. It will thus be seen that Dr. Allinson's allegations, quoted above, are " not founded on fact, nor supported " by anything except his own dogmatic assertions.

In the following pages it will be seen that I have set forth, somewhat at length, the arguments and proofs briefly summarised in the preceding paragraph, which go far towards demonstrating the correctness of that portion of the " fruit and nut theory " which asserts that cereals are an unnatural and unwholesome food for man. Oddly enough, in the issue of the *Weekly Times and Echo* just preceding that from which the above quotation was taken, Dr. Allinson furnishes still another proof that cereal foods are unnecessary and unwholesome. I quote :

" The value of milk as food is that it contains its nourishment in an easily digested form, and those who are used to meat and wish to adopt a non-flesh diet will find the free use of milk very helpful whilst making the change. Sickly, weak, and delicate persons w ll find milk a valuable food if they will use it as I advise, and growing children may take it freely, but only at meal times. When babies cannot get breast milk, then that of the cow, mixed with barley-water, must be given. Breast-fed children, when weaned from the bosom, must be allowed milk and bread, or milk and some farinaceous food. As children grow older they may still use milk freely ; at meals they should drink it mixed with water instead of tea and coffee. They may also have porridge and milk, or brown bread and milk sop, at least once a day. Grown-up persons will also find milk puddings advantageous.

" During illness or recovery from disease I find milk an invaluable food. In disease of the stomach and bowels I rely almost entirely on milk and barley-water to keep my patients alive, whilst the necessary curative changes are proceeding. In ulceration of the stomach a diet of milk and barley-

either boiled or baked; or they may be cooked in water at scalding point until the yolk is hard, but the whites not leathery. To return to the consideration of Dr. Allinson's prescription, it will readily be seen that, if cereals are so difficult to digest that they must not be used in illness, it will surely be a good idea to see how a non-starch diet will work after recovery.

The fact that the whole civilised race is making cereals the basis of food will be seen to be no proof that these foods are not harmful. In arguing against the use of spirits, tobacco, tea, and coffee, I have often had the fact pointed out, with a triumphant gesture, that Mr. Smith or Mrs. Brown is eighty (even ninety) years old, and has used some one or more of these poisons all his or her life. Temperance reformers and hygienists have shown that such instances have been in persons of exceptional vigour, and in spite of the harmful effects of these poisons; and usually such aged persons have exceptionally good habits to compensate for the alcohol, tobacco, tea, or coffee. *Eating too much* is a common source of a shortened and decrepit life, and *moderation in the quantity of daily food* is usually found a characteristic of the aged poison user. This is pointed out in this connection only to emphasise that law is universal, and is always in force; the laws of physiology are as exacting as the law of gravitation; and whoever habitually takes poison, or indulges in any pernicious or unwholesome habit, shortens life, and suffers resultant decrepitude; and the fact that the poison user sometimes reaches the age of ninety is more an argument that man's natural term on earth is 120 years, than that the tobacco, or coffee, or whiskey does no harm. The same is true of the universal custom of eating bread. Plato tells of a nation where the men had no gray hairs at a hundred years; that they usually reached a great age; and that the men were frequently fathers of children after the age of a hundred. If one arguing in favour of bread could show such a nation, using cereals, it would be a conclusive proof that this food is not much, and probably not at all, harmful; but it will be found that such records are always of a people who do not use bread. On the other hand, the fact that illness is wellnigh universal points to a univeral cause; and the purpose of the following pages is to point out some of the proofs of this position.

It is quite true that many individuals reach middle life (or what is usually called that) habitually using bread and cereals, and in apparent good health; but the race must be run before anything is proven. In my childhood I knew a neighbouring farmer who used to make daily trips, in the severely cold winters of northern Pennsylvania, to a village a half-dozen miles away, without any coat and without other clothing than the shirt he wore in summer time. The team which he drove hauled heavy loads of wood, and this necessitated a slow pace, and the teamster followed at a slow walk. He laughed at the foolishness of his neighbours who coddled themselves in coats ; and, strangely enough, he got on for years in seeming good health. Ultimately he lost his health, and died in middle life ; but, while in seeming vigour, his case was no proof that his habit was not injurious ; it was proof only that the powers of his system were able for a time to overcome, and not at once die from exposure. During the civil war in America, it was found that farmers' sons did not make as tough and enduring soldiers as the young men about the towns, who had been clerks in stores, and like employments, where there was less strain, and less exposure to the extremes of weather, than had fallen to the lot of the farmers. This was a great surprise ; most persons would have supposed that the fresh air and out-door work of the young farmer were more favourable to health and endurance than the coddled life of the town boy. When it came to the test, the only explanation of the failure of the farmer is in the supposition that the daily struggle with trying winter weather gradually undermines the vital powers of the system. Just so, I think, it is with starch foods ; they are, like the inclement weather of our northern winters, an unnatural and health destroying strain upon the vital powers ; and, while the vigour of youth and middle life is sufficient to overcome the strain for a time, it is only for a time ; broken health and premature decrepitude are sure to follow.

This explains the phenomenon of the milk and water diet. When a person is stricken with illness, and vitality at a low ebb, it has been found by most physicians of all schools that milk is the best food, and that cereals—and especially bread—must be left off. When the usual vigour of the system has been established, the patient is again able (apparently) to endure the accustomed strain of starch foods. When my Pennsylvanian farmer was taken ill, his common sense forbade his exposure, in insufficient clothing, to the strain of severe winter ; after the usual vigour had been re-established, he was again able (apparently) to endure the strain of his accustomed exposure.

When I began the Vegetarian life, some eight years since, I had neuralgic headaches, coming on periodically about every three weeks, of so severe a nature that I was compelled to take to my bed for a day ; and the headache was not appeased until after several paroxysms of severe vomiting. I had inflammatory rheumatism, which sometimes sent me to bed for a week or two at a time. I had lumbago, of such a nature that I could stoop only with great difficulty at my best, and was sometimes unable to walk for days at a time. I inherited a tendency to skin cancer ; and my face was habitually inflamed and pimpled. Have had chronic sore eyes since boyhood ; and for twenty years preceding the adoption of Vegetarianism my eye-balls and eye-lids were at all times inflamed ; and I usually felt an impulse to screen their lamentable condition from the gaze of others. Upon the adoption of Vegetarianism my health greatly and rapidly improved; the redness disappeared from the eye-balls and largely from the eye-lids; the rheumatism greatly improved; I was in every way better. But one serious difficulty from which I all my life have suffered (since the age of twelve) was not appreciably improved. I quite universally experienced a heaviness from one to three hours after meals; an inability to work and repugnance for any needed labour, and especially for mental work. I suffered much from heaviness and drowsiness, and could only with great difficulty bear a dull discourse; and in the evening, after my usual dinner, it was often quite impossible to keep awake. I have often, at such times, pulled hairs from my head (and I have none to spare!) in an attempt to pay some regard to the decencies required by the situation.

Some three years ago I was loth to discover, but forced to admit, that no progress was being made; indeed, I perceived that I was losing ground, and came to the conclusion that the roseate view I entertained as to a virtual restoration to health was doomed to disappointment. I was in this condition and this frame of mind, like many others, when I concluded (in September, 1889) to try what a non-starch dietary would do for me. I sensibly improved from the first week's trial. I had often noticed, previously to the trial of the non-starch diet, knowing I was to be called upon for mental work soon after a meal, that if I took a slice of brown bread— a tenth or a fifth of what the needs of my system required—I escaped the hateful heaviness, while at the same time the small amount taken was sufficient to appease hunger; and I had often for years wished that I might be able to eat as much food as the needs of my body required, and at the same time feel as delightfully free from the dreaded drowsiness as when eating only a sandwich. I had not gone a week on the new diet, until I discovered I could eat a full meal, and if desirable proceed at once to the transaction of business, or the writing of an essay, without any sense of having eaten, and without the slightest heaviness or drowsiness. I now average about seven and one-half hours of sleep in the twenty-four, as against about eight and one-half on my former cereal diet; and whereas then I was quite given to feel dull in the evening, and very apt to fall asleep if subjected to the infliction of a dull discourse; now I am wide awake until midnight, or later if occasion requires; and I am entirely freed from any fear of the somnolent effect of the dullest discourse. It was the freedom from the heaviness resulting from sluggish digestion that was noticed at the outset. As weeks and months wore on, I found distinct improvement in the rheumatism that had not—under the Vegetarian diet —entirely disappeared; now for some months I have been wholly free.

As already stated, I have not been free from lumbago for thirty years. While the first period of my Vegetarian diet had greatly benefited this infirmity, latterly I had found myself losing ground. After some months of the new diet, I found the lameness gradually disappearing ; now, at the end of nine months, although still far from well, I find myself apparently as much improved as by all the years devoted to a Vegetarian diet.

One swallow does not make a summer ; and, although at the time of writing I know of a score or more of persons who have been benefited—some of them most signally—by the non-starch diet, I do not claim that this demonstrates anything ; but I urge this fact, taken in connection with the array of evidence briefly set forth—in many cases merely hinted at—in the following pages, as a good and sufficient reason to justify all persons, at all out of health, in giving this system a thorough trial.

There are some considerations regarding the putting of this matter to a practical test, to which I wish briefly to allude. It will be seen, in the quotation from Dr. J. Milner Fothergill, in the following pages, that that deservedly noted physician strongly advised the pre-digestion of starch foods, not only for infants, but for many adults as well. This starch food, when converted into soluble sugar, is used for supporting the heat of the body, and also the vital energy. It escaped the observation of Dr. Fothergill that the dates and figs of the South, cheaply and abundantly supplied by our markets, are loaded with this identical soluble sugar, so much sought after. I find that a liberal supply of such fruits, taken in connection with an equally liberal portion of the watery acid fruits of the North, distinctly lessens the amount of nuts, or milk, eggs, or cheese, that will be required for adequate nourishment.

One important advantage, from the adoption of the non-starch diet, is sure to be realised alike by the Vegetarian and the non-Vegetarian. Bulk is an indispensable element in carrying on healthy nutrition ; it is well known that a horse needs something more than grain and water, although these contain every element of nourishment ; some hay, or straw, or chaff, must be added. The cereals and vegetables used by all civilised races afford this necessary bulk. When these foods are omitted from the dietary, it will be found that all persons will at once reach out for something to take the place ; the result will be a large consumption of fruit where little or none was taken before. It will be found that this is a great gain. There is much less tendency to eat too much than when eating cereals, and if too much food is taken less damage is done than by over-eating of cereals.

The greatest possible gustatory satisfaction is given by a diet of fruits, nuts, milk, eggs, and cheese ; and there will be found less temptation towards cooking and the highly seasoned compounds which are prime factors, alike in the Vegetarian and the non-Vegetarian diet. Indeed, an earnest seeker after simplicity in diet will find that there is nothing so conducive to unwholesome cooking as the starch foods. The proof of the pudding is in the eating—a trial of the non-starch diet will confirm the correctness of my claim. I fearlessly assert that cereals and starch foods, on the one hand, and intricate cookery and luxurious compounds on the other, mutually play into each other's hands ; and whenever and wherever the non-starch diet is adopted it will be found that the tendency is all the time towards simplicity and healthfulness. At the same time, a noteworthy feature is found in the fact that—owing, no doubt, to the more perfect nourishment of this diet—less craving for variety will be experienced on it than on any other.

A non-Vegetarian, any one accustomed to the mixed diet of the world, will find quite as much advantage in this diet as the hygienists and food reformers. Although partaking of fish, flesh, and fowl, it must be remembered that still the cereals and starch foods form the basis of the usual dietary ; and an elimination of the starch foods therefrom will at once relieve many of the ills by which all persons are quite universally more or less affected. While it is quite true that flesh is an excremental, irritating, and more unwholesome food than milk, or eggs, or cheese, still it has one distinctive advantage over these foods—there is less tendency toward constipation. Whenever the flesh-eater can be persuaded to adopt the non-starch diet, he is sure to find all the advantages enumerated above ; and then, as elsewhere remarked, finding that there is a great scientific truth at the bottom of the food question, there will be a decided tendency, on the part of these converts to the non-starch diet, to give up flesh-eating altogether.

Since this anti-cereal food crusade has attracted some attention, I have been besieged by letters from persons asking for specific directions as to the amount of eggs, and milk, and cheese needed in a diet for an adult. This of course depends upon the habits, labour, exercise, and condition of the individual, and the only general rule to be given is to eat as much of fruit and nuts as is easily digested and is distinctly demanded by the appetite ; and to use only so much of the animal products as may be needed for the adequate support of the system, seeing to it that the digestive and excretory organs are fully able to take care of, and dispose of that which is eaten. For several weeks, upon first commencing this diet, I ate an abundance—all my appetite craved—of apples and acid fruit, a few nuts, and an average of six eggs per day ; at this time using no milk and cheese. I walked three or four miles a day—not enough ; a man engaged in manual labour would have needed more nitrogenous food. On this diet I felt no longing whatever for other or forbidden articles of food, and whoever has such longings may be sure he or she is not well fed.

Had I taken the dates and figs freely, the accustomed acid fruit, and three or four ounces of almonds, Brazil nuts, walnuts, and the like, I am hoping that two or three eggs per day would have been adequate. However, I have been for years more accustomed to fruit-eating in large quantities and can relish daily considerable quantities of dates and figs ; those beginning on this diet, and less accustomed to fruit must use more milk and eggs —always managing to use enough figs and tart fruit (and if an invalid distilled water) to keep the bowels open.

The following letters, taken from the (London) *Weekly Times and Echo*, are inserted here because of the practical light thrown on the question of what foods should be taken by those who wish to give the non-starch food system a trial.

SIR,—I have read with pleasure the interesting letter, under the above title, of Mr. George Poyntz in your last issue. Because nuts and fruits are expensive, and the best varieties well nigh out of the question in England, Mr. Poyntz recommends a diet of meat (fresh aud tinned), milk, eggs, cheese, and dried preserved fruits, with the chance use of fresh fruits and nuts when plentiful and cheap, using water only as a beverage.

I wish to remind Mr. Poyntz that eggs and cheese are less expensive— for a given amount of nourishment—than even tinned meat, and that these foods take the place, and perform every useful service, of animal flesh, and are free from the excremental and injurious element necessarily found in every piece of muscular flesh. The function of the blood is twofold ; it carries nourishment to the tissues, and absorbs and carries from the working tissues the oxidised and broken-down tissue—the ashes, so to speak, of the system—and this broken-down tissue is discharged daily (or ought to be) through the bowels, kidneys, and skin. If a bullock is killed to-day, and a portion of the red meat eaten, there is, inseparable from each minutest portion of the flesh so eaten, an excremental substance which, if the animal had not been killed, would have been discharged from the bowels in a short time, and such food is not appetizing, when one comes to think of it, even if we have become accustomed to the enormity. If Mr. Poyntz will follow the diet he has laid down for himself I am quite sure he will find his joints better, together with other substantial improvements. He will be less liable to feel heavy after eating, or during a dull discourse; he will feel distinctly lighter, freer, more buoyant, more vigorous, more capable of work, and especially mental work But he can accomplish all this on fruits—with eggs, or milk, or cheese—whichever agrees best, and is most easily digested. Milk is apt to be " heavy," hard to digest, and constipating (it is always safest to boil it), but those who had not been able to use it with a mixed diet, and where the vital powers were overtaxed, in the protracted and difficult digestion of bread and cereals, have had no trouble where all starch foods are dropped and a plentiful supply of fruit substituted. And this is true of those who have found eggs or cheese difficult. Learn to eat large quantities of fruit, to let all bread stuffs alone, and difficulties vanish. I buy the mildest and least salted cheese to be obtained, and then have it cut in thin slices, warm water poured upon it, and allowed to stand until it begins to soften; then pour the water off, and heat the cheese until melted. It is afterwards just as good cold as heated; but this process takes out much of the salt, and freshens and sweetens—the disagreeable taste much is less pronounced. Eggs have the advantage of containing even less earthy matter than beef or mutton; and both eggs and melted cheese (as above) are more easily digested than beef or mutton, unless the latter are thoroughly minced by a machine. Animal flesh is such an unnatural food for man, that it not only has to be modified by cooking, but it ought to be artificially masticated as well by mincing.

Mr. Manning, in his admirable letter in same issue of *Weekly Times and Echo*, suggests that perhaps we are better with an abundant supply of fresh fruit without nuts or animal products. I fear that everyone who tries to sail on this line is sure of shipwreck. If we could get an abundant supply of bananas cheaply, there would be less fear, for bananas are about twice as rich as wheat in muscle-making nourishment; whereas the fresh fruits of this climate—valuable for their water, acids, and relish—are substantially without nitrogen, that necessary food for muscle so abundant in some varieties of nuts, and in eggs, milk, cheese, and animal flesh; and whoever tries to live on an exclusive diet of such fruit will find himself living off and consuming his own tissues; and even if bananas are added, and the necessary nitrogen furnished, I am of opinion that there would still be found a longing for fat—in my opinion a necessary element in man's food—and if not supplied in nuts, the natural source, or eggs and cheese, the best substitute, there will be running off after some form of the fleshpots that contains this necessary element. Rash hygienists and Vegetarians, unacquainted with the necessary elements of human food, have done themselves and others irreparable harm in persisting in the use of an inadequate diet. A plenteous supply—not a gorge—of all needed elements of food is an indispensable requisite for health. Starvation is very unattractive to the practical minded, and an exclusive diet of northern fruits is on the borderland.                                 EMMET DENSMORE, M.D.

---

Sir,—In your last issue, Mr. J. Hayward quotes from Dr. John Edward Morgan the statement that when bread is properly masticated and insalivated that a part of the starch in the bread is converted into soluble sugar. It is quite true that a mouthful of bread thoroughly mixed with saliva will show a trace of sugar when tested; but it is also true that a mouthful of bread, masticated as thoroughly as Mr. Hayward would esteem practicable, has but a small portion of its starch converted into sugar, as any good chemist will demonstrate when required. All physiologists agree that the gastric juice neutralizes the action of the saliva; and when these facts are borne in mind it will be seen the great bulk of the starch foods, even after thorough mastication, must wait until the intestines are reached before digestion (preparation for assimilation) proceeds.

It is quite true that those persons who have to pay considerable attention at times to mastication get on much better when they insalivate their food than when they bolt it; but there are two reasons that may account for this fact, aside from the process of converting insoluble starch into soluble sugar. One is the certain fact that people do not eat as much food when thoroughly masticated as when the food is hurriedly swallowed; and again, food which has been thoroughly masticated in the mouth requires much less peristaltic (or churning) action of the stomach, and consequently much less strain upon the vital force. Furthermore, bread and the starch foods are so naturally repugnant and distasteful taken dry (or even with sultanas, as Mr. Hayward recommends), that nearly all persons will come at last to softening their bread with some liquid or goody, and then insalivation is out of the question. I have spent years in teaching myself and trying to teach others to properly masticate food; and when successful, the results have not been gratifying—not more than the lessened quantity of food and the greater ease of digestion, because making the food fine before it enters the stomach, will easily account for. And even if the fullest possible insalivation would greatly mend matters (the contrary of which I confidently maintain), it will be found much easier to teach people to do without starch foods altogether than to induce them to properly masticate their food. Mr. Hayward tells us that if bread is eaten anyhow, and washed down with some liquid, it becomes the "staff of death." The outlook must be discouraging to Mr. Hayward when he reflects that hygienists, in England and America, for twenty-five years have been trying to teach the importance of thorough mastication, and no appreciable headway has been made. It is because progress—so it seems to me—does not lie in that direction.

The poet Shelley, in discussing the food question, made a very practical and common-sense suggestion. He urged that it is folly to be for ever arguing out this question when a few months' practice will settle it. It is for a trial that I plead. Let any invalid try the thorough mastication of starch foods for a few months, and watch results. Then try a diet of fruit and nuts, supplemented with eggs, or milk, or cheese—whichever agrees best—and mark results. So far, all who have tried this course are enthusiastic in its praise.

Bulk is a very necessary element, and when starch foods are not used, a large quantity of fruit is sure to be eaten. This is at once a great gain; as fruit opens the portals of the system—a most important matter—and abounds in cooling and purifying acids.

It is my hope and expectation that when this diet is adopted by Vegetarians they will be able to hold what they gain, and not lose as many converts in the summer as were made in the preceding winter's compaign. Furthermore, the anti-cereal food doctrine appeals as strongly to those who are not Vegetarians as those who are; when the whole people can be induced to substitute fruit and nuts for bread, cereals, and vegetables they will note such marked improvement that they will see the food question is fraught with great importance; and when they begin earnestly to study food, it will be seen that flesh meat is excremental and unwholesome, that milk, eggs, and cheese are in every way more desirable; and then Vegetarianism will make real progress. EMMET DENSMORE, M.D.

———

Sir,—I have received a letter from a working tradesman stating that after a month's trial of the non-starch diet he has felt obliged to give it up far a time on account of severe constipation. He writes : " Although I do not abate my confidence in all you advance in regard to the cereals, I think you will probably see fit to modify somewhat the extreme regime to working men and others, to whom more than a pound of fresh fruit is beyond pecuniary means. Everything has gone on satisfactorily until within two days. Stiffness of joints disappeared, cheeks filling out and more colour (they tell me so), hearing improved, and more activity. By the way, last Sunday I walked upwards of fifteen miles to see the old mother, altogether without a headache, which has never happened before. So far so well. The warning of costiveness nature gave was unheeded, and feeling hungry took a feed of strawberries, milk, and figs. I devoured altogether that day about six eggs, rather hard boiled, but well masticated. Digestion all right, but in the evening commenced my troubles." My correspondent then gives the particulars of a constipation which was so severe that he felt it wise to return to a moderate amount of cereal food.

It will be noted that the improvements testified to are somewhat extraordinary ; and are gimen that has brought such signal benefits ought not to be lightly given up. Mr. Manning, Vanbrugh-hill, S. E., has been securing for friends 20lb. boxes of dried figs, of good quality, at 3d. per pound. A ten-gallon carboy of distilled water (exclusive of carriage) can be obtained at Apothecaries' Hall at 3d. per gallon. A pound of these figs stewed in two or three parts of distilled water, with a pint or more of stewed gooseberries (which if stewed in a double boiler need no addition of water) would have made for my friend five or six pounds of wholesome and nourishing food at an expense of sixpence. Of course, with the warning nature gave him, he ought not to have eaten six eggs in a day ; but, even after the damage has been done, if he had tried this fig and gooseberry food (and the equivalent of the gooseberries in some other acid fruit when these are out of season), to resort to, and had used no other food for a day or two, he would have found his hunger appeased, his strength renewed, and his constipation overcome. As soon as the bowels are at work again restore the eggs, or cheese, or milk to the dietary gradually. In a few days he would have been able to eat his usual amount of eggs and fruits, have performed his usual amount of work, and would have found the improvement in his health stalking ahead.

Let it be remembered that wheat in some regards is an ideal food. It contains all the elements of nutrition (except free oil—in my opinion, an indispensable element) in about the needed proportions ; and whoever makes wholemeal bread the basis of daily food, and has yet remaining enough vital force to digest and assimilate this food, is well nourished. Moreover, the fine particles of bran set up a daily inflammation in the bowels, and for years insure a daily movement. It does not matter to the victim that this daily inflammation is slowly but surely laying the foundation for a permanent derangement of the entire digestive tract, and that the great expenditure of vital force needed for the digestion and assimilation of bread is gradually but surely undermining the nervous system—the fact remains that the person is nourished, and not constipated ; a most important desideratum. When anyone excludes bread and starch foods from their dietary they are apt to find two stumbling-blocks in their path ; they are apt to be constipated, and apt to rely too much on watery fruits, and suffer from lack of nourishment. I explain to all that it is of the utmost importance to be well nourished, and to have a free action of the bowels. Since the nuts we can get in England (to say nothing of expense) are hard to assimilate by our bread-enfeebled digestive organs, and since the fruits of northern climates are lacking in essential (especially nitrogen) elements of nutrition, I advise that eggs, milk, or cheese be freely taken ; and since these foods are of a constipating tendency, especially where the stomach and intestines have for years been inflamed by wholemeal bread, I advise that large quantities of fruit be taken daily. With these facts and principles in view it ought not to be difficult for any earnest intelligent person to escape both the Scylla and Charybdis—the constipation and lack of nourishment—of the anti-cereal food regime.

I do not claim that this changing from a life custom is an easy matter, or that it is without difficulties. It it neither. But I do claim that any person who will earnestly and persistently pursue a diet of fruit and eggs, or milk, or cheese, with or without nuts, for a time, is sure of such reward in improved health and lengthened days as is beyond my power adequately to express.

EMMET DENSMORE, M.D.

---

As elsewhere remarked, I have valued the arguments set forth in Dr. De Lacy Evans' "How to Prolong Life" more as confirmatory of the position that starch foods are calculated to undermine the nervous system, and so make way for all kinds of diseases, than as a system of itself fitted to persuade people at once to forego the use of cereal food ; indeed, it is taught by Dr. Evans that all cereals ought to be wholly relinquished only after middle life. As confirmatory of the teachings of Dr. Evans, I insert a newspaper clipping, just received by a Vegetarian friend, from Buenos Ayres, South America ; and I also wish to point out that the experience and the present views of Dr. Alanus are as much an argument against the usual mixed diet as against that of the Vegetarian—differing only in degree :

A DREADFUL BLOW TO VEGETARIANISM.—AN EMINENT PARTISAN REPUDIATES IT.

Vegetarianism all over the world has received a severe blow. Its most zealous scientific partisan in Germany—its most quoted learned authority, the writer of so many leaflets and polemical pamphlets—Dr. Alanus, sends the Vegetarians his farewell :—"Warum ich nicht mehr Vegetarisch lebe," (Why I no longer live as a Vegetarian), such is the title of an article sent to the Rhenish *Courier* by Dr. Alanus. The former preacher of the vegetable diet writes : " Having lived for a long time as a Vegetarian without feeling any better or worse than formerly with mixed food, I made one day the disagreeable discovery that my arteries began to show signs of atheromatous degeneration. Particularly in the temporal and radical arteries this morbid process was unmistakable. I could not interpret this symptom as a manifestation of old age, and being furthermore not addicted to drinking, I was utterly unable to explain the matter. I turned it over and over in my mind without finding a solution of the enigma. I, however, found the explanation which I had sought so long quite accidentally in a work of that excellent physician, Dr. E. Monin, of Paris. The following is the verbal translation of the passage in question :—' In order to continue the criticism of Vegetarianism, we dare not ignore the work of the late lamented Gubler on the influence of the vegetable diet on the chalky degeneration of the arteries. Vegetable food, richer in material salts than that of animal origin, introduces more mineral salts into the blood. Raymond has observed numerous cases of atheroma in a monastery of Vegetarian friars, amongst others that of the prior, a man scarcely thirty-two years old, whose arteries were already considerably indurated. The naval surgeon Treila has seen numerous cases of atheromatous degeneration in Bombay and Calcutta, where many people live exclusively on rice. The vegetable diet, therefore, ruins the blood vessels and makes one prematurely old, if it be true that man is as old as his arteries." It must produce at the same time tartar, the senile arch of the cornea, and phosphaturia.' Having seen these newest results of medical investigation confirmed by my own case, I have as a matter of course returned to a mixed diet. I can no longer consider purely vegetable food as the normal diet of man, but only as a curative method which is of the greatest service in various morbid states. Some patients may follow this diet for weeks and months, but it is not adapted for everybody's continued use. It is the same as with the starving cure, which cures some patients, but it is not fit to be used continually by the healthy. I have become richer by my experience, which has shown me that one single brutal fact can knock down the most beautiful theoretical building."

———

Vegetarians ought to realise that an article like this, first printed in German, and having such vitality that, six months after, it is circulated in English in South America, is well calculated to do Vegetarianism great harm ; and I maintain that the policy of ignoring such matters, and of refusing to discuss them, helps on the damage by giving the impression that Vegetarians have no answer. Indeed, so far as I know, except the theory that nuts and fruits are the natural food of man, and that all starch foods are disease inducing, there is no answer to Dr. Alanus. Dr. Allinson's reply, published in the *Vegetarian*, to the effect that first he had seen very little atheromatous degeneration among Vegetarians, and second, that he had seen much more among the eaters of a mixed diet, will be seen to be no answer. It is quite natural that there should be more cases of this disease outside than within the ranks, when we consider that there are but a few thousand Vegetarians, and millions who are eating a mixed diet ; and especially when we consider that cereal and starch foods form the basis of the mixed diet, And this leads to the consideration of another most important fact. If Dr. Alanus abandons Vegetarianism because cereal food has thickened the walls of his arteries, is he not still in danger, since the cereals are yet the basis of his food ? It will be seen that the only logical deduction from the experience of Dr. Alanus is that cereal foods must be wholly abandoned, if we are to be entirely free from danger. It is quite true that heretofore, without the key which is supplied by the following pages, Vegetarians are in greater danger than mixed feeders ; but it is a difference only of degree ; and when we bear in mind they use considerable portions of eggs, milk, and cheese, and have used only a little more of the starch foods than others, we see they are in but little more danger.

An earnest appeal is made to the Vegetarian and meat-eater alike, to put the anti-starch food system to a practical test. From Her Majesty the Queen to the lowliest of her subjects, and in my own land from the most influential President to the most humble citizen, there is a bond of sympathy— the greatest of earthly blessings, health. The Vegetarian is interested, not only to be made free from the danger of illness, but in a system that removes the stumbling-block from the path of that movement that has a a clean life, and the avoidance of inflicting suffering upon animals, so much at heart.

But to the meat-eater, this question is not less important. To prove the correctness of the claim herein set forth, all that is necessary is at once to abstain from all bread, cereals, pulses, and starch foods. When obtainable, it will be found advisable to substitute liberal portions of dates, raisins, and figs for the accustomed bread. Continue the usual portions, if you prefer it, of fish, flesh, and fowl. Apples also take the place of bread, and a little practice will enable all persons to relish their accustomed meat, or fish, or eggs, as well with apples as with bread ; and whenever dates and figs, or fresh apples are not obtainable, other fruits will be found entirely adequate. Dried apples and prunes are always to be had ; and a diet of meat, or fish, or eggs, liberal in quantity, and abundance of stewed apples or prunes, will accomplish wonders in the way of restored health, unstiffened joints, improved complexion, buoyant vigour, and freedom from the heaviness, sleepiness, and tired-out condition of the bread-eater.

I urge the reward of full and perfect high health, lengthened life, and increased happiness, with usefulness to each individual ; but there is yet another consideration. My readers, I trust, will agree with me, that if the system put forth in this little book is based in truth, it is fraught with tremendous import to the human race ; and each one of us who may give this regimen an adequate trial, not only finds a rich reward in individual gain, but also has the satisfaction of helping to make known this most important discovery. I appeal to every reader to lend a helping hand. Let us band together, prove all things, hold fast to that which is good, and do what we may to usher in the day so beautifully pictured by the prophet-poet, Shelley :

" Mild was the slow necessity of death ;
The tranquil spirit failed beneath its grasp,
Without a groan, almost without a fear ;
Calm as a voyager to some distant land,
And full of wonder, full of hope as he.
The deadly germs of langour and disease
Died in the human frame ; mild purity
Blessed with all gifts her earthly worshippers.
How vigorous then the athletic form of age !
How clear its open· and unwrinkled brow ;
Where neither avarice, cunning, pride, nor care,
Had stamped the seal of grey deformity
On all the mingling lineaments of time.
How lovely the intrepid front of youth !
Which meek eyed courage decke l with freshest grace ;
Courage of soul, that dreaded not a name,
And elevated will, that journied on
Through life's phantasmal scene in fearlessness,
With virtue, love, and pleasure, hand in hand.

   .      .      .      .      .      .

O happy earth ! reality of heaven !
Thou consummation of all mortal hope !  .  .  .  .
   .      .      .      .      .      .

Of purest spirits thou pure dwelling place !
Where care and sorrow, impotence and crime,
Langour, disease, and ignorance, dare not come,
O happy earth, reality of heaven ! "

# The Natural Food of Man.

By Emmet Densmore, M.D

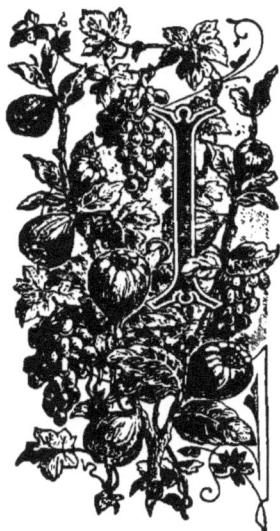

I USE the word natural, in the sense of God-designed. I am one of those unfashionable scientists who perceive design in the universe. It does not matter what title we give the Supreme Ruler: Natural Law, or God, or what you will: there seems to me conclusive evidence of intelligent design in the Great Artificer. The mechanism of the human body—the exquisite adjustment of means to ends—has been the wonder and delight of the anatomist and physiologist since science began. A man-made pump or engine manifests design; the human heart, while incomparably superior as a piece of mechanism, is no less the result of design. In meditating upon this subject, it has occurred to me that the Divine Architect, in contriving the several organs of the human body, has necessarily adapted that organism to a procurable food; that there is at hand a food for man exactly adapted to the needs of his organism; and it is in this sense that I use the term natural food.

We observe that all animals below man are supported by food spontaneously produced. Moreover, the careful observer of Nature will notice that those animals, and birds, and fishes, which are subsisting on foods spontaneously produced, are quite universally in perfect physical health and vigour. It has occurred to me that God is no respecter of persons, and that in all probability he has provided a food as well adapted to the needs of man's organism as he has for the needs of the lower animals; and that man has only to solve this riddle, to find his natural food, and to learn to obey the laws of his being, to banish sickness from the race.

Since all other animals subsist on food spontaneously produced by Nature, it is fair to conjecture that primal man must also have subsisted on such foods. It is affirmed by naturalists, from a study of the nature of man's organisation, that his birthplace must have been located in a warm climate ; hence we ought to look to the products of the South, in our search for man's natural food. It has seemed to me probable, if primal man subsisted on foods spontaneously produced, that those same foods are so produced to this day. In conjecturing as to what those foods must have been, it is well to bear in mind that primal man had no tools, and that without tools he could neither slay animals nor catch fish with any regularity or reliability. It must also be recollected that fire and cooking are the result of subsequent discovery, and without fire it is plain that man would not subsist on animals, even allowing he could catch them, if he could find foods at hand less repulsive. Are there such foods ? The nuts and sweet fruits of the South are yet the most toothsome and delightful food that we have. Are those foods an adequate nourishment for man ? Years ago, when I first began the investigation of this subject, I was aware that fruits abounded in carbonaceous elements, but was under the impression that for the needed nitrogen we must look elsewhere. I was much gratified, upon further investigation, to learn that some fruits are very rich in nitrogenous elements ; the banana, if reduced to the same state of dryness as wheat, has rather more than double the proportion of nitrogen, and is fully equal in this regard to the pulses. Upon further investigation I learned that nuts are not only rich in carbonaceous food, but some varieties are also richer in nitrogen than any of the cereals ; indeed, it will be found that the simple products of nuts and sweet fruits abound in all the needed elements of human food, and that they have these foods in the needed proportion, as determined by chemical analysis.

A sceptic at my elbow reminds me that it does not follow, even if it be admitted that nuts and fruits were the food of primal man, and if on this food primal man was as free from rheumatism and other diseases as the birds and animals—it does not follow that these foods are an adequate or desirable food for civilised man ; that perhaps generations' of civilisation have changed his nature, and that his habits and methods of life in civilisation demand a different food from what he needed in barbarism. A scientific mode of determining this question is to make the experiment. I have determined to try it ; in the meantime, I desire to make some observations, and to offer some suggestions.

When I first caught a glimmer that perhaps nuts and sweet fruits are the natural and adequate, and only desirable, food of man, I was enabled to find a solution of some problems that had greatly perplexed me. In the practice of my profession, in an attempt to wean my patients from the diet of civilisation to a hygienic and Vegetarian diet, I had been struck by the persistence with which nearly all people cling to sweets. In all civilisations we find sweet confections and desserts. It at once occurred to me that if sweet fruits are an important part of man's natural food, and if in his journeyings on earth he has strayed out of reach of those foods and learned to live on flesh and cereals, that this persistent demand for sweets is an effort on his part to get a needed food from which he has unwittingly been deprived. The key of nuts and sweet fruits enabled me to understand the universality of our habits of sweet desserts and candy eating.

In weaning patients from the usual to the Vegetarian diet, I pondered much upon the tenacity with which the races of men cling to oily foods. I was never able to understand the problem of why the negroes of the South so persistently demand bacon with their hominy. With this new-found key, I can see that, if nuts are also a necessary portion of man's natural food, and if in his journeyings he has been and is deprived of this food, then his substitution of milk, butter, and fat meat, may be explained as a persistent demand of his bodily needs to get a lost but much needed element of food. I can see that, after all, the impulse to eat bacon with hominy may not be so far out of the way.

For years a Dr. Salisbury has been astonishing the thinking members of the medical profession in this city by a repetition of wonderful results from his methods of practice. Dr. Salisbury's treatment is largely dietetic ; and, whether his patients be obese or emaciated, the food is the same—all the lean beef the patient can eat, and all the hot water he can drink. To the emaciated, or to those not obese, he allows the addition of as much butter with the beef as may be desired. For food and drink, beef and hot water—absolutely nothing else. Let it be observed that this food is free from starch. I was reminded, in meditating upon this, that my natural foods for primal man—nuts and sweet fruits—are also free from starch.

The physicians of Europe have been greatly astonished at the marvellous cures performed at certain institutions, commonly known as "The Grape Cure." I have read that at these institutions the patients are given all the grapes that they desire to eat, and absolutely no other food. It is my intention to verify this report ; if it be a fact, it is significant. I am reminded that in this food there is no starch. I have read also of similar cures, called "Milk Cure," "Whey Cure," and "Cherry Cure." Absence of all starch foods is a feature in all these institutions.

In meditating upon this subject, I said to myself : But starch is a good food for cattle and horses ; and, pursuing the subject, I could see that very naturally it is so, since all our cereals are at the outset grass seed, and the Great Designer would not make animals calculated to subsist on grass that would not also be prepared to use the seeds of grass. Many years ago, when I read of Vegetarians who had become very radical in diet, and who were making experiments on raw wheat, I was unable to conjecture how the wheat could be obtained in its best estate for eating raw. American green corn is most palatable when the grain is in the milk ; and one can easily strip our large ears of maize of the husk, and it is quite a palatable food eaten raw ; but to procure the grains of wheat in this state always presented a difficulty. It occurred to me that, since grass is the natural food of cattle, it was easy to see that to the ox or the horse this presents no difficulty ; and I began to have a suspicion that perhaps wheat and rice, and the cereals generally, being only grass seed, are the natural food for cattle, and not for man. Straightway I remembered that one of the greatest difficulties I have in the treatment of dyspeptics, is to get their stomachs able to digest bread. Even if the wheat and meal were baked in the form of "gems," entirely unleavened and unfermented, the difficulty seemed quite as great ; also, if the wheat or oats be simply boiled, it is still very difficult food for many stomachs to digest. In our own practice, we had found it necessary to use a large proportion of milk with the bread ; we found many patients whom we carried triumphantly to a surprising degree of bettered health on an exclusive diet of brown bread with milk, but whom we were unable to manage on a diet of bread and fruit, excludng all animal foods. At the time, I accounted for this fact by conjecturing that the digestive organs had been weakened by long generations of meat-eating, and that, although wheat forms a large proportion of the best food for man, he, from lack of exercise and the resultant vigour, has become too feeble to digest it. If, however, it will finally be made clear that the cereals (only grass seed) are the natural and desirable foods for cattle, but are not adapted for the digestion of man, there will be developed another explanation.

For years Mrs. Densmore and myself made a speciality of the reduction of obesity, and the treatment of chronic diseases resulting from weakened and disordered conditions of the digestive system. We early saw and affirmed that obesity and emaciation are different expressions of the same difficulty; that they are each the result of a diseased and weakened state of the digestive apparatus. True, given foods, as bread and potatoes, are instrumental in creating excessive weight in individuals ; but we were reminded that usually men and women do not become obese until after forty, and the foods which in middle life rapidly create obesity, are eaten at twenty and twenty-five years of age with impunity. Hence we saw that it is not the food, so much as the state of the system. In emaciation we saw patients eating large quantities of nourishing foods, only to continue to emaciate, the same patients, early in life, had been able on the same foods, and in less quantities, to keep up a full quota of flesh. We early saw that obesity and emaciation spring from a common cause ; and, since I have had my suspicions aroused that perhaps starch foods, while excellent for cattle, are not good for man, I have meditated further on this subject. It is quite universally known, by physicians and laymen alike, that the greatest promoters of obesity are bread and potatoes. The thought occurred to me that if starch foods are the cause of obesity, and if obesity and emaciation spring from a common cause, we have another hint that starch foods may perform an important part in laying a foundation for all the diseases of the digestive tract. Every thinking and candid hygienic physician must have been surprised at the occasional spectacle of patients who had tried for months, and even years, to live on cereal foods and fruits, who had made indifferent success, and who appeared to be much benefited upon a return to a flesh diet. I have seen instances of this at various times during the last twenty-five years, and have been greatly perplexed by it.* If it shall transpire that starch is an unnatural and undesirable food, it will help to solve the problem.

When Mr. Banting first published his letters, giving the world the benefi

---

* I noticed in the *Vegetarian* of January 18th, page 46, a communication referring to Dr. Alanus and his withdrawal from Vegetarianism. If your readers will read that account carefully, they will see a confirmation of my position, namely, that many earnest Vegetarians have seen evidences of failure in following out the rules laid down by Vegetarians. There are many reasons for suspecting that atheromatous degeneracy of the arteries is due to the use of cereals and starchy vegetables.

of the system by which he had been freed from superfluous flesh, and his health greatly improved, they gave great prominence to the idea that fats and oily foods are productive of obesity. A few years since, Dr. Ebstein, of Germany, promulgated the doctrine that it is starch and sweets that create obesity, and not oils. Indeed, he instituted a cure for obesity, which consisted largely of fat meat. Experimenting with Dr. Ebstein's system, Mrs. Densmore and I verified largely his claim ; we found that it is starch, and not oils, that creates obesity ; moreover that, if all starchy foods are rigorously eliminated from the diet, a considerable quantity of oily substances can be taken with impunity, and a reduction of flesh go on. This is one point in favour of the theory that fruit and nuts are the natural food of man, and not calculated to create any disease. When the oil is eliminated from nuts, the remaining portion is chiefly nitrogenous.

Meditating on the question of obesity, and the uses of fat in the animal economy, I am able to see that Nature provided the bear with a large share of adipose tissue, with which he goes into winter quarters, hibernates during the winter months, and comes out in the spring emaciated, but vigorous. I also see that cattle fed on grass in the spring and early summer, during the late summer and early autumn, in a state of nature, are fed in addition with grass seed, loaded with starch, as part of their food. The result of large quantities of starch in this grass seed is seen in the storage of large quantities of fat in the bodies of the cattle. This seems to be a provision on the part of Nature against the inhospitable winter, and enables the cattle to withstand the cold weather and inadequate supply of food, where, if it were not for the storage of fat provided in autumn, the animal would be unable to live through the winter ; while, with this fat, it comes out in the spring " spring poor " as the farmers say, but vigorous, and much in the same condition that the bear does after hibernation. Squirrels, mice, and other animals, are provided with an instinct that prompts them to store away nuts in the autumn, on which they are able to subsist in the winter. And it appears, theoretically, not only that wheat and rice and all cereals are the natural food for cattle, but that their tendency to create obesity is a wise provision of Nature, to enable the animal for whom it has been provided to withstand the inclemency of our winters. But men, born in a warm climate, where fruits are ripe the year round, and where there is no winter to withstand, need no provision for laying up a periodical store of fat ; and hence man's natural food, nuts and fruits, have no tendency to create obesity. Moreover, it is easy to see why, in accordance with this theory, starch foods are wholesome and proper for cattle, and disease-producing in man.

In the treatment of some hundreds of patients for obesity, Mrs. Densmore and I noticed that wonderful cures of patients suffering from neuralgia, rheumatism, severe and long-standing headaches, nervous prostration, and many serious ailments, followed our treatment ; while, except a simple herb-tea cathartic, no medicines were used ; the treatment was dietetic, and consisted in taking away all bread, cereals, and starchy vegetables, and giving them flesh foods, and non-starchy vegetables. I have asked many Vegetarians to explain, from a Vegetarian standpoint, this surprising phenomenon ; and, so far, no one has responded. If it shall some day be proven that nuts and fruits are the only scientific and allowable food for man, and that the cereals, while wholesome for cattle, are disease-producing in man, an explanation is found.

This theory, that nuts and fruits are the God-designed food for man, explains the failure of so-called " Edenites," in California, and of advanced Vegetarians the world over, who, having an instinct that cooking is an unnatural preparation of food, have tried to take their food raw. Not having this theory, that nuts and fruits are the only allowable food for man, they have taken it for granted that wheat and the cereals are the natural food, and attempted to eat these in the raw state. I have not been able to learn of any single individual, much less a community, who has succeeded for any considerable time in living on raw grains. If the cereals —cattle food—are unnatural for man, we can easily understand why cooking may be as necessary, to prepare them for human food, as it is to make meat palatable. I am of opinion that the instincts of man will reject raw wheat and raw pulses almost as surely as raw flesh; and the fact that the process of cooking is necessary to render the cereals palatable is as much an argument against them, as the fact that cooking is necessary for flesh is an argument against flesh foods.

The processes of Nature are harmonious, and her changes are gradual. It has always seemed strange to me that Nature provided us with milk as our natural food for the first year of life, and that, after we pass the period during which milk is our natural food, we are suddenly confronted with so great a change as bread. While attending medical lectures, I was struck with the assertion, on the part of the lecturer on physiology, that the nearest imitation there is for milk is ground-almonds and water; he affirmed that that mixture has a milk-like colour, and that it is scarcely distinguishable chemically from milk. Since getting the hint that very likely fruits and nuts are the natural food for man, I can see that it requires no great change for the child to leave off milk, and to take, instead, fruits and such nuts as are scarcely dintinguishable from milk. I have made no experiments and no researches; but I conjecture that it will be found, upon analysis, that cows' milk is as like the elements of food contained in the grass, as human milk is like ground-almonds and water. The scientists of to-day are making great efforts to get a healthy drink for man. We not only transport spring water from one end of the planet to the other, but go to great expense in the distillation of water (distilled water being said to be the ideal drink for man). Any one who will live exclusively on nuts and fruits will find that they are provided in fruits with water distilled in a finer laboratory than man yet knows how to make, and that he needs no other drink.

All farmers and horsemen are aware that, while their horses are kept the year round in a stable, and fed largely on dried grains and dried grass, they are very liable to be constipated; but it is also quite universally known that as the same horses are turned out to grass, in fact as soon as they are put upon their natural food, the constipation vanishes. It is logical to expect that, if we are usually fed upon unnatural diet, there will be great tendency to constipation in the human family; and also to expect, if we ever ascertain what is meant by natural food, and put ourselves upon it, that then, as with the cattle on the grass, the constipation will speedily be overcome. I believe it will be found, with all persons who will live exclusively on nuts and fruits, with such eggs and milk as may be necessary in the absence of an abundant supply of the best nuts and sweet fruits, that the constipation will be speedily and wholly overcome. This is a matter the importance of which can hardly be too much dwelt upon. Constipation is the bane of modern civilised life. Dr. Abernethy's three rules for health are : "Keep the head cool, keep the feet warm, and keep the bowels open." When that food is found which is absolutely and scientifically adapted to man's organism, constipation will be impossible.

The cocoa-nut and the banana afford more food to the acre than can be obtained from cereals. I am told by a friend—but I have not yet verified it—that Mr. Buckle, in his "History of Civilisation," affirms that an acre of ground devoted to nuts and fruits will support about sixty people, whereas, devoted to wheat, it will only support two or three. However this may be, it is undeniable that the earth will produce far larger quantities of food in nuts and fruits than in cereals, and the food so obtained is procured with less labour and expense. Almonds, raisins, and other nuts and sweet fruits, outrank all other foods in gustatory pleasure. These foods, unlike the cereals, need no addition of salt or sugar to make them palatable. This is as would be expected upon the hypothesis that these foods are scientifically adapted to man's use. Cattle, on the contrary, have the utmost relish for the cereals without sugar or salt, which is an evidence that these are the natural foods for them. Cattle fed monotonously on cereals preserve the keenest relish ; I am satisfied, from experiments lately made, that man fed monotonously on fruits and nuts will preserve as keen a relish and appetite as the horse fed on oats ; a thing unknown to the modern eater of flesh and starch foods.

I have been, from time to time, much interested in the writings of Mr. Hills in favour of raw foods ; at the same time, my instinct rebelled against his suggestion that even the pulses may be better raw than cooked. In my opinion, the weakness in his position is not in the idea that raw foods are best for man, but in taking it for granted that the pulses are a natural and proper food. I learned, while pursuing medical studies, that starch foods are distinctly better cooked than raw, for the reason that the envelope containing the starch granules is broken in the process of cooking, and therefore made digestible and assimilable. But this reasoning does not apply to nuts and fruits. To a normal appetite and stomach, nuts and fruits are distinctly better relished raw than cooked, and more easily digested and assimilated. A milk diet, especially for invalids, has grown in popularity throughout civilisation for years. If the underlying thought of this paper shall be proved correct, it will easily be seen that the popularity of a milk diet is the result, not so much of its own excellence, as that by the exclusive use of it the patient is freed from the injurious effects of cereals and starch.

There has been a great deal of difficulty for Vegetarians to give an adequate explanation of why it is that the meat eating Englishmen and Germans are of a larger stature, and have distinctly more vigor, than whole races of people in India, China, and Japan, who live almost exclusively on cereals ; but if it be true that all starchy and cereal foods are ill adapted as the food of man, and require a far greater expenditure of nerve force and vitality in digestion than is needed for natural foods, then it will not be difficult to understand why the rice eating people are dwarfed and less vigorous. It is the teaching of naturalists, that the longevity of animals is about six times the age required for maturity. Even under the stimulus of modern life and foods, twenty years is about the average age at maturity. Genesis says : "And his years are a hundred and twenty." Men and women who live to the age of seventy, eighty, and ninety years, are yet thirty, forty, and fifty years short of their natural term. The rice eating people of the East do not use flesh foods, and as a consequence do not suffer from rheumatism and the acute diseases so abounding in Western civilisation; but they are dwarfed and weak, and have no greater longevity. If it shall be proven that the cereals and vegetables are an unnatural and unnecessary strain upon the digestion, and drain upon the vital forces, it will explain why those people, with their simple cereal foods, are no longer lived than the Western civilisee.

Nuts and sweet fruits are eaten with no salt, and no seasonings, and no cooking ; flesh foods and cereals quite universally require cooking, and salt, and other seasonings. Cereals lead to cooking, cooking to seasoning, seasoning to stimulants, and stimulants to undermining the nervous system —to morbidity and death. Morbidity, disease, and premature death, will be seen to be as universal as starch and stimulants. Are these conditions the inevitable consequence of the use of cereals as food ?

# Part II.

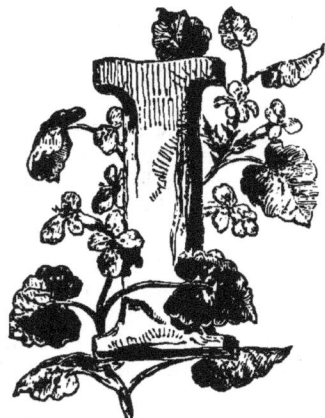

I N a former issue of the *Vegetarian*, I gave an account of some experience and experiments that occurred in a medical practice for the reduction of obesity, and asked the following question : " Why is it that signal benefits are pretty sure to follow in great multitudes of patients where no other treatment is given than confining their food to animal flesh, and such fruits and vegetables as have no starch, excluding potatoes and all cereals ? " It will be observed that the reduction of obesity has nothing to do with the question ; nor did, nor does, it follow that other physicians and experimenters may not have had similar results in exclusive feeding of meat to patients who are affected with other diseases than obesity. If it be true that an exclusive diet of the flesh of animals is frequently attended by a marked and sometimes permanent gain in the condition of patients long and seriously out of health, it is a subject demanding the most earnest and painstaking investigation on the part of Vegetarians, and food reformers under whatever name.

Since writing the essay entitled, " The Natural Food of Man," recently published in the *Vegetarian*, I have for the first time read a book entitled, " The Relation of Alimentation to Disease," by J. H. Salisbury, A.M., M.D., LL.D. Dr. Salisbury is a member of the Philosophical Society of Great Britain, of the American Antiquarian Society, of the Natural History Society of Montreal, of the American Association for the Advancement of Science, etc., etc., and is a scientist and microscopist of some note. I am thus particular to note the standing of this author, in the hope that food reformers will give some earnest attention to the important and remarkable claims put forth by him   I quote from the preface of his book :

" In 1849 I began the study of germ diseases. Those of plants first occupied my attention ; afterwards, those in animals, and in man. I had previously been engaged in the exact sciences of chemistry, botany, geology, zoology, and mineralogy. In 1846 I was appointed assistant in the Chemical Laboratory of the New York State Geological

Survey, and in 1849 I became Principal of the Laboratory. I had been a graduate of Albany Medical College, and in 1850 I entered upon the practice of medicine.

"I was immediately and forcibly struck by the almost entire want of medical knowledge in regard to the true causes of disease, and by the consequent uncertainty that must and did exist as to the means of combating and curing pathological states. This uncertainty hampered me at each step of my practice. The art of Therapeutics was a chaos whose sole order consisted in dealing with established pathological conditions as though they were the disease itself, rather than what they actually were, viz., consequences based upon antecedent and obscure states arising from an unknown cause. In consumption, for example, this want of thorough and basic knowledge conduced to our treating certain abnormal states as inflammatory, when they were in reality paralytic ones, as I shall demonstrate in subsequent pages.

"The grim list of so-called 'incurable diseases,' and their steadily increasing death-rates, riveted my attention and fascinated my thought. I attained an entire conviction that they must be curable ; that, since abnormal conditions could be established in previously healthy organisms, their causation must be discoverable ; and that the mind of man must be endowed with sufficient power to trace the interlinked sequences of disease back to their primary source. I determined to accomplish this discovery, if possible, before my exit from this world. I started without theories, without prejudices. I had no beaten rut to confine me. I resolved to collect and sift actual facts ; to the ultimate testimony of these alone I looked for a solution of the riddle. . . .

"In 1854 the idea came to me, in one of my solitary hours, to try the effects of living exclusively upon one food at a time. This experiment I began upon myself alone at first. Fortunately, in our works on Physiology, beans are placed at the head of the list of foods as regards their nutrient qualities. On this account I opened this line of experiments with baked beans. I had not lived upon this food over three days, before light began to break. I became very flatulent and constipated, head dizzy, ears ringing, limbs prickly, and was wholly unfitted for mental work. The microscopic examination of passages showed that the bean food did not digest ; that it fermented and filled the digestive organs with yeast, carbon-dioxide, alcohol, and acetic acid ; that the sacs of legumen containing starch granules were insoluble in the digestive fluids, and consequently these fluids could not reach the starch until it had fermented and liberated sufficient gas to explode the sacs. By this time the starch was too far changed into gas, alcohol, and vinegar, to afford much nourishment to the body.

"From this date until September, 1856, I subjected myself to testing upon my own person the effects of exclusive feeding upon several other foods in turn, as often as I could find time to do so. My eyes opened to the vast reach of the field before me. I had found a door standing ajar, through which I began to get glimmerings of light in the right direction.

"In September, 1856, I hired six well and hearty men to come and live with me, as I myself would live, on baked beans. This experiment and its results are fully described further on. In 1857 I engaged four other well men to live with me upon oatmeal porridge solely, for thirty days. That experiment is also given in detail hereafter. In 1858 I took nearly 2,000 hogs, in separate lots and in different pens, so that I might test various modes of feeding them, and carrying my experiments on to the death-point, as could not be done with men. In order to be sure of my data, I tended, fed, and dissected them myself ; it was not work that could be done with kid-gloves on ! These experiments also are fully given in subsequent pages. Later on I employed men from time to time to live with me on other kinds of food, one kind at a time ; some of the results of such living are duly given under their proper headings. By 1858 I began to understand from what cause all our diseases eminate, excepting those arising from injuries, poisons, and infections, and to hope that the day was not far distant when I should be able to cure them. . . .

"Having satisfied myself as to the causation of disease, my next step was to complete a therapeutic system which should meet the facts in the case, and obtain the end in view— that of combating a pathological groundwork by removing its cause, and thus effecting a radical cure. The publication of this work in its entirety has been delayed over twenty years, in order that sufficient cures of so-called 'incurable' maladies might place both discovery and method of treatment beyond all reasonable doubt. Hundreds of cures now attest to their utility, not alone in my own practice, but also in that of other physicians of high repute, both here and in England."

In the fifth line of the first chapter of Dr. Salisbury's work is a noteworthy statement : "*Improper alimentation is the predisposing cause of disease.*" Near the close of the volume, from a long chapter detailing the particulars of the treatment and feeding of the 2,000 hogs referred to in the preface, I quote further :

"From these experiments we learn this important lesson : *even hogs cannot 'make hogs of themselves' with impunity, on a diet that their digestive organs were never made to properly digest and assimilate.* The structure and functions of the digestive apparatus, in each class of the animal kingdom, determine its natural and healthy food. Upon this alone can it live without producing disease ; upon this it thrives, and if discreetly fed it escapes all those fatal chronic maladies which arise from long-continued abnormal alimentation.

"This fact is so vital, nor alone to animals, but also, and in even greater degree, to . Man, that I may be pardoned if I repeat, in closing my work : *Nearly all the diseases that 'flesh is heir to,' aside from those produced by parasites, poisons, and injuries in general, are the terrible outcome of defective and unhealthy feeding.*

"With the mass of evidence herein presented, I may safely rest my case for the time being, content with having called thoughtful attention to a great but much ignored truth. It is my abiding hope that the people may be brought to see these facts for themselves, and may, by individual and intelligent self-control, restore and maintain the oft-imperilled balance of health. Without it there is neither beauty, use, nor happiness for us ; in its absence, all the great glories and truths fade away from our sick vision. If we will not learn Nature's methods, she crushes us in the reversion of her laws, and passes on. But if we examine and inaugurate her processes, we become as calm and as strong as she, and, like her, in our lives we receive and manifest the Divine."

The chapters of Dr. Salisbury's book detailing the particulars of the feeding of himself and several healthy labouring men, first upon an exclusive diet of baked beans, and subsequently upon an exclusive diet of oatmeal porridge, make startling reading for Vegetarians. I quote from pages 184 and 191 :

"In September, 1856, I engaged six strong, healthy men, in the vigour of life, ranging in age from 25 to 40 years, to feed upon a special line of diet solely, with the understanding that I would pay them $30 per month each, if they submitted faithfully to the rigid discipline laid down. At the same time I explained to them the kind of food upon which I should require them to live, and the exercise and other regulations marked out. All thought the diet and drinks could be easily endured—in fact, enjoyed—especially as they would have no manual labour to perform. They all entered upon the undertaking with the feeling that they would have a fine time at my expense. The diet consisted, first, of baked beans and coffee. This to continue for one month, or until otherwise ordered by me. Exercise to be a two-mile walk, morning and evening. To retire at nine p.m. and rise at six a.m. Drinks between meals, cold water. . . .

"In October, 1857, I placed four hearty, well men upon oatmeal porridge as an exclusive diet. It was seasoned with butter, pepper, and salt. Cold water was drank between meals, and a pint of coffee, seasoned with sugar and milk, was taken with each meal. The men were the most healthy and vigorous I could procure. All regarded themselves as perfectly well, and none had ever suffered any severe illness. Their ages ranged from twenty-three to thirty-eight years. I required them all to live with me continually night and day, and to take no food or drinks other than what I gave them. They were to receive $30 per month each, with board and lodging. I subjected myself to the same rules and regulations, asking of them nothing but what I would and did do myself. This gave them a confidence and pride in the work, each striving to outdo the other in the strict observance of the rules."

It must be borne in mind that Dr. Salisbury aimed to get a more rapid effect than would have followed if he had given these men only a needed amount of food, and with an endeavour to preserve their health in as good condition as possible. On the contrary, he desired to have them eat all that their appetites would permit, with a view of hurrying up whatever conditions would naturally ensue. According to the memorandum which Dr. Salisbury published, they were bloated and constipated from the third day. A daily report of each is given; I quote samples from one. On the 6th, one of them experienced dizziness, a ringing of the ears; on the 9th, "ears ring, dizzy, hands and feet prickle"; by the 13th, "ears ring, reel in walking, confused"; on the 18th, "feel numb all over, weak at times, walk with difficulty, feet drag." I quote from pages 187 and 188:

"Symptoms of progressive paralysis, or locomotor ataxy, began to show themselves in all six cases on the tenth day. These paralytic and peculiar symptoms increased each day after the tenth. On the sixteenth day the disease was so marked, that not one of the six could walk straight without support. All wobbled and dragged their legs, not being able to lift them clear of the floor. . . . .

"My boarders, on the 19th morning, all presented such a forlorn, dilapidated appearance, that I feared I should lose my reputation as a caterer, and also all my guests, unless I changed my diet list. They had all lost heavily in weight, and were much debilitated.

| " A weighed 138 lbs. | Loss in 18 days | 22 lbs. |
|---|---|---|
| B  ,,  116 ,, | ,,  ,, | 29 ,, |
| C  ,,  136 ,, | ,,  ,, | 19 ,, |
| D  ,,  143 ,, | ,,  ,, | 23 ,, |
| E  ,,  147 ,, | ,,  ,, | 25 ,, |
| F  ,,  126 ,, | ,,  ,, | 22 ,, |

"When, on the morning of the 19th day, I set before them nice beef-steaks, freed from fat and white tissue, they were all greatly delighted, and ate ravenously of them. I gave to each ten ounces of meat, with a good cup of clear coffee. Beef seasoned with butter, pepper, and salt; no other food or drinks. At dinner gave each twelve ounces of beef-steak, prepared as for breakfast, and half a pint of clear tea. The meal was hugely enjoyed.

"All now began to breathe easier and to feel clearer about the head. Passages less frequent, though still large and numerous. During the afternoon, all were in a state of enjoyable relief, and were ready to speak a good word for their host and his house."

Dr. Salisbury relates that on the 20th and 21st he gave them three meals a day, chiefly of beef-steak, and discharged them on the 22nd day, feeling in good trim. The outcome of the experiment on feeding on oatmeal exclusively is reported to be similar. On the 30th day he changed their diet to broiled beef-steak three times a day. His patients at once showed marked signs of improvement, and were discharged on the 34th day "well and happy."

It is not so very strange that a number of men, accustomed to active exercise, can be placed upon an exclusive diet of baked beans or oatmeal, and, by following this persistently for twenty or thirty days continuously, eating much more than the system requires, should develop serious symptoms of ill-health ; but it must be confessed that it *is* strange that these symptoms should be overcome by a few days' continuous feeding of three hearty meals of beef-steak, with no other food. It is to be regretted that Dr. Salisbury does not give more particulars as to the amount of food the men consumed at each meal, or at least each day ; and moreover, in the interests of science, it would have been well if he had given the names and addresses of his " boarders," and had procured from each a sworn statement of the facts, followed by the name, address, and statement of the notary before whom the depositions were made. But an important fact is open to the world, and easily verified. It is this : Dr. Salisbury conceived that most diseases arise from eating improper foods ; and that, instead of entirely and easily digesting and assimilating, giving health and strength, the great bulk of the foods used in civilisation ferment in the stomach and intestines, causing gas, flatulency, inflammation, failure of digestion and assimilation, resulting in inadequate nutrition, a prostration of the nervous system, and a general break-down, and terminating in the hydra-headed brood of modern diseases. He claims to have proven by experiments that all cereals, vegetables (in the common use of that word), and fruits, if used exclusively and continuously as human food, result in intestinal fermentation, ending sooner or later in loss of health and a general break-down ; that the muscular tissue of beef, separated from fat, gristle, skin, and connective tissue, used exclusively and continuously as human food, does not ferment, and is readily, easily, and perfectly digested and assimilated; and that two to four pounds of beef per day, with no other food whatever, and with three to six pints of hot water daily taken as he directs, with no other liquid, and with a cathartic sufficient to cause a daily movement of the bowels, is universally followed with great benefits to all, and usually with the fully restored health of the patient. On this system he commenced the practice of medicine, making a specialty of so-called " incurable " cases, and specially of consumption, tumours, etc., together with all nervous diseases; he began that practice over thirty years ago, in a western city ; after a score of years of great professional success, he came to New York some ten years ago, and he had such phenomenal success in this city as to attract attention abroad. A few years since he established in London a branch office or centre from which the Salisbury treatment is given ; and a most noteworthy product of the London centre is a book published by a patient of Dr. Salisbury, a remarkably brilliant and able writer, entitled, "What Must I Do to get Well" (Elmer Stuart). This lady has filled her book with eloquent and enthusiastic praise of the treatment to which she feels she owes her life. Speaking of Dr. Salisbury, she says:

"By 1858 he perceived clearly and unmistakably that all *diseases not caused by accident, poisons, or infections, eminate from unhealthy alimentation.* And, having at last reached the cause, the remedy was not far to seek. His life mission opened itself out fully before him ; and earnestly, and with a deep sense of responsibility, did he set about it—not so much to make a living for himself, as to help others to live—to prevent disease, and to cure it. Nobly has he fulfilled that mission, as hundreds can now testify, who but for him would to-day be taking their long sleep in 'the land where no man dwelleth,' or would be as I was, hourly, for eight and a half most weary years, sleepless, helpless, barely able to move, and night and day unceasingly suffering great anguish. If you who read these lines had but seen me then—could but see me now, after a few short months of the diet and hot water ! Two months and a half after I began the strict treatment, I could bend, and put on my shoes and stockings, and lace and unlace my boots, which I had been unable to do for nearly ten years. And then, gradually, each invalid appliance and device, and all cushions, etc., were discarded ; and oh, the *heartfelt* joy with which I saw the last of these nuisances disappear ! "

Further on, Mrs. Stuart says :

"I was desperately ill when I began the strict Salisbury treatment ; I wish I could describe how ill, and with what complications, in which most severe gout and rheumatism, contracted muscles and rigid joints, acute neuralgia all over me, dyspepsia and insomnia, each in an aggravated form, played its evil part ; but I have gone right ahead ever since, gradually but steadily on the mend, with no disheartening relapses. I see no doctors, take no medicines or stimulants, only stick to hot water and the minced beef diet."

Some months since I excited a veritable hornet's-nest about my head by asking in the *Vegetarian* the question, "Why is it that an exclusive diet of flesh is often attended with remarkable and sometimes with permanent gain in health ? " My own answer to this enquiry is, that cereals and starchy vegetables are a natural food for cattle, but not for man ; that, when used continuously as human food, they sooner or later undermine the vital force, prostrate the nervous system, and prepare the way for the appalling scourge of universal illness and premature decrepitude that afflicts all civilised peoples. I will risk ostracism on the part of my brethren in food reform, by calling special attention to the following quotation from page 103 of Mrs. Stuart's book :

"And in this place, with all possible earnestness, I entreat and solemnly warn you, especially if you are ill or any way ailing, never to allow yourself to be ensnared by that calamitous blunder, that gigantic fallacy, *Vegetarianism*. Of all the gratuitous modes of flinging away precious health and inducing illness, this is about the foremost for rashness and folly. I speak from experience, for, regarding it as the ideal humane and perfect diet (I still consider it all that, only, unfortunately, there is lacking to us the *ideal stomach* necessary for its digestion and assimilation), I anxiously desired to follow it always, and, to my life-long repentance, tried hard to do so six separate times, beginning more than eleven years ago. I carefully studied all its literature on which I could lay hands ; I corresponded with and implicitly obeyed the guidance of some of its leaders, with this result—that twice I brought myself so near death's door that I heard the hinges creak, and, still undaunted by that dire experience, tried it yet four times more, causing myself very serious illness. And but that I had, to begin with, an iron constitution, nay an adamantine one, this wretched diet—unnourishing, because fermentative, flatulent, impossible of digestion and assimilation—would have had me long ago under, instead of on, the green earth. I never yet knew a Vegetarian, and I have known many, possessed of much real stamina. He may keep well by dint of hard labour, or brisk exercise and careful living all round, for a while—even for a long while, I admit—but when illness does overtake him, *having no reserve of strength*, down he runs like a clock with a broken mainspring, and his resisting and rallying force, thanks to his inadequate nutrition, is lamentably weak. It may be 'economical,' as some count economy, penny-wise and pound-foolish ; but the bill is high in the end that we pay, with doctors' fees and lost health. A 'navvy' or a coal-porter may stow away and be able to digest and work off the regulation amount of peas, beans, lentils, oatmeal, etc. ; but for us, more or less sedentary beings, there are many far cheerfuller and more seducing ways of upsetting our stomachs, if we must do so, than Vegetarianism ; and few—I speak feelingly—are more dangerous, chimerical, or so idiotic."

I will venture but one more quotation from this remarkable book ; but I am free to confess that I esteem it a rare treat of wit and wisdom from beginning to end ; and if I were permitted, wherever Mrs. Stuart recommends beef and hot water, to substitute nuts and fruits, and, in the absence of the right varieties of nuts and fruits, to substitute for beef and hot water milk and eggs (and fasting) and hot water, I would recommend it as *par excellence* the best guide to health with which I am acquainted. I quote, beginning on page 154 :

" I now come to a point which, though I have before alluded to it, I beg your leave to urge once more upon you *strongly*. Indeed, there are two points, and from experience and observation I hold them both to be of great importance. First, I advise any one suffering from sleeplessness, neuralgia, gout, rheumatism, indigestion of all kinds, including sleep-walking, cramp, nightmare, sensations of falling, and so on, and from delicate health generally—even if such persons persist in rejecting the *strict* diet—while taking their hot water daily, as often as they can manage it, to make their *last meal at night a meat meal entirely*, preferably of beef broiled, roasted, or minced, according to their illness, and their powers of mastication and digestion. And even those in comparatively fair health (especially those of us not growing younger) would be very wise to make the lean meat, roast or broiled (which includes fish, poultry, and game) their *chief* food of an evening ; *because* the digestive powers, in nearly all cases, are weaker at night than at mid-day, and the lean meats digest very quickly and readily, and do not produce distention and flatulence, as other foods are apt to do. The evening meal, while hearty, should be the lightest of the three. It is, further, very bad for 'the wind,' by which I mean the respiration, to go to bed either on a full stomach, or on one containing an undue amount of fermentable food, such as bread, puddings, etc. A great deal of so-called asthma, even in young people, owes its origin to this latter pernicious practice. Let any one try this meat supper conscientiously *for a week or two consecutively*, and he will experience a wonderful benefit. The gouty, and rheumaticky-gouty, will find, as a result of a moderate entirely meat meal at night (not forgetting their hot water, of course), that they are able, among other good things, helpfully and less and less painfully to use their poor weak hands in the morning, and several advantages will accrue in the other cases also ;

and even yet more abundantly will the gain be felt (almost at once too) by the *sleepless*. I am now morally certain of this, that very many severe illnesses, in both the young and the elderly, owe their origin solely and entirely to a superfluity of fermentable food and drinks at late dinner—too much bread, vegetables, sweets, fruit, etc., probably all together, *in undue proportion*. Then almost imperceptibly begin wakeful, restless nights.

"From my own experience I can fully bear witness that the sleeplessness due to fermentation is altogether a most distressful sensation, and makes one far more wretched and uneasy than even that produced by too strong tea. The unconscious victim of fermentation soon has recourse to drugs and sleeping draughts, which cannot remove the cause, but instead increase the evil; for complications will ere long arise, indigestion, constipated bowels, feebler health and resisting power, etc., until it ends in a complete break-down. I am speaking from my own *closely observed* experience, for I can now prognosticate pretty accurately my night's rest from my supper. With people who are in fairly good health, it is not what they eat *occasionally* that can hurt them. It is a continual dropping that wears the stone away—the continuously and persistently eating the wrong food at the wrong time, in the wrong proportion, that causes the final disaster. I know not who invented the stupid saying that bread is the 'staff of life,' so often hurled triumphantly at me in the sanguine expectation of its discomforting experience and fact. Whoever it was is as answerable in one way for the world's unhappiness, as Solomon is in another, whose dictum respecting the rod and the child made of my childhood a misery at the time, and a pain to look back on. But Solomon had more excuse for his aphorism, since with such a large family he must often have been driven nearly distracted, and constrained to lay about him with lavish profusion. Tea being the cup that 'cheers but not inebriates,' is another moonshine proverb."

If my Vegetarian friends will bear with me for this seeming heresy, and for calling marked attention to these remarkable utterances, I promise them before the close of this essay to show some physiological and philosophical grounds for my position; and that, while the flesh of animals is undoubtedly an excremental, poisonous, unnatural, and unwholesome food for man, still the "Salisbury Treatment" is a stubborn fact in the world, and is a valuable milestone in the path of progress, helping to point out the colossal mistake the race has made in adopting for food those cereals and vegetables which require to be cooked in order to be digested and assimilated, and which, in the very nature of their ill adaptation to the human organism, are an ever present cause of nervous prostration and its resultant evils.

As to the cause that produces diabetes, physicians are quite undecided. But they are united upon this, that all cereal and starchy foods ought to be prohibited the patient. Quain's "Dictionary of Medicine," one of the latest and best received old school authorities in England and America, says: "All authorities agree that meat should be the chief constituent of the patient's food, and that starch and cane and grape sugar should be avoided, as well as all those foods containing them." To quote further from this authority: "Haricot beans, peas, and all cereals, tapioca, sago, arrowroot, all forms of macaroni, cheese, potatoes, carrots, turnips, parsnips, and beet-root, are on the forbidden list."

Quain tells us that a variety of food is very desirable, and proceeds to give quite an elaborate list of articles that may be allowed the patient. If one takes into consideration the great damage that is usually done to patients by old-school medication, the fact that they are almost universally ignorant of the remedial value of hot water, and considering also the relatively large variety of foods which are allowed the patient, one does not wonder that this authority states that diabetes is a very serious disease, and is almost never considered curable. A method of treatment quite largely adopted in America by practitioners in various schools of medicine consists chiefly in confining the patient's diet to skimmed milk only, from four to eight quarts being recommended in the twenty-four hours. As might be expected, this system of treatment is far more successful than that recommended by Quain, and usually adopted by the old-school practitioners.

Dr. Salisbury recommends a very radical treatment, and reports a very great success. In addition to the hot water usually prescribed to patients, he allows beef-tea made from pure lean meat fibre, and for food confines the patient to the muscle pulp of lean meat. After giving minute directions as to the hot water, beef-tea, beef-pulp, and hygienic directions, Dr. Salisbury remarks, on page 129 :

" By judiciously and persistently following out the foregoing plan of alimentation, treatment, etc., the diseased organs and system generally soon begin to take on a more healthy state. The urine contains every succeeding day a smaller proportion of sugar ; its density lessens steadily, its quantity decreases ; the colour heightens, the appetite improves, the eyes grow brighter and brighter, the skin gradually loses its dryness and becomes more soft and oily, and the mucous membranes less and less feverish and dry ; the thirst ceases, and the entire organism takes on, little by little, yet certainly and surely, the actual appearances, states, and conditions of health.

"In less than one week's time, after this treatment is thoroughly entered upon, the quantity of urine decreases from gallons to about two quarts per diem ; and the density falls from 1040 to 1060 down to 1026 to 1034, varying with the advancement and severity of the disease. The thirst usually ceases in about three days, after which the sufferings of the patient are comparatively slight.

" The least deviation on the part of the patient from the course marked out can be at once detected by the watchful and expert physician. A single mouthful of bread, vegetables, fruit, sauce, sugar, or any fermenting farinaceous or saccharine food, will elevate the density of the urine many degrees, by increasing the sugar in it, and the quantity voided will be much greater. The physician should be able to perceive immediately any departure of the patient, and call him to strict account. No one need hope to handle this disease successfully, without an unfaltering observance of the foregoing rules and regulations."

Further on, Dr. Salisbury says :

" To effect a cure, we must cut off (as far as possible) all food which goes to make animal sugar. This includes vegetable food, animal fats, tendon and connective or glue tissue and cartilage. Also all excess in drinks. Abstinence in these respects will lessen the labour of the diseased parts, and by degrees subdue their excessive activity. Normal states then ensue ; and if these are well established for a few months, and accompanied by appropriate medication, they break up the diseased habit and restore normal conditions, which, becoming in their turn permanent, finally and thoroughly cure the disease."

It will be seen by this that Dr Salisbury esteems diabetes a surely curable malady. But how does he accomplish it ? Precisely by those means, in my judgment, which cure diabetes under the skimmed-milk regimen, and that sometimes effect a cure under the old-school treatment: by the elimination of all starch foods from the dietary. Now, when we consider that diabetes is never developed except in those persons who are accustomed to a starch dietary; that, under the old-school treatment, diabetic patients are always helped, and sometimes cured, by partially refraining from starch food; and that, under the skimmed-milk treatment, these patients are frequently cured, and under the strict Salisbury treatment quite universally cured—is it not fair to conclude that diabetes is caused by a diet of cereals and starch foods?

A large business is done in America in the preparation and sale of foods for infants and invalids. It is proclaimed in the literature of the various firms that these foods are quite free from starch: that this substance has been converted into soluble dextrine by pre-digestion. The late Dr. J. Milner Fothergill, of London, was a very successful physician, an able writer, and a painstaking student. From a pamphlet entitled, "Nutrition for Infants and Invalids, with Suggestions from J. Milner Fothergill, M.D.," I quote:

"Gentlemen,—Having requested me to give you my opinion, as a food expert, upon your 'Lactated Food,' I do so herewith. You state that it contains 'the purified gluten of wheat and oats, with barley diastase and malt extract combined with specially prepared milk sugar'; in other words, that it is self-digestive as regards the conversion of insoluble starch into soluble dextrine and maltose. My experiments with it lead me to hold that this is correct. When lactated food is placed in water hot enough to be sipped, a rapid transformation of the starch remaining in it (by the diastase it contains) goes on; and a nutritive fluid is the result, which requires but a minimum of the digestive act. The resort to farinaceous matters, pre-digested, must become greater and greater as our knowledge of digestion and its derangements waxes greater. It is not merely in the case of feeble infants that such pre-digested starch and milk-sugar are indicated and useful; persons of feeble digestion require these soluble carbo-hydrates, which they can assimilate."

I desire to call attention to the last two sentences of this remarkable utterance. Dr. Fothergill tells us that we must resort to the pre-digestion of farinaceous foods as our knowledge of digestion waxes greater. I ask food reformers to carefully consider whether it will not be better to avoid using those foods that require to be "pre-digested." I doubt not that generations of feeding upon a food which is physiologically ill adapted to the human organism—namely, the cereals and starchy vegetables—will result in multitudes of persons of such feeble digestion that they are unable longer to assimilate this food, unless a resort be made to pre-digestion and artificial aid.

Perhaps the most convincing proof of the claim, that all cereals and starches are unfit for human food, is found by a reference to the physiology of digestion. The human stomach is supplied with a digestive fluid that readily prepares nitrogenous and albuminoid foods for sanguification and assimilation. The function of the stomach is not only to liquefy and make fine; but, when the right kinds of food are furnished to it, it also prepares these foods for assimilation, and that process goes forward at once. When the cereals and starch foods are eaten, the gastric-juice neutralises the effect of the saliva, and the only effect accomplished is to liquefy and make fine, and pass the contents on to the intestines, where the pancreatic juice and intestinal solvents are able to prepare the starch for assimilation—for available nutrition. The gastric-juice is able to neutralise the saliva, but is powerless to render the cereals assimilable. In the meantime hours have been consumed in the process ; and greater nerve force has been expended than is required to digest and sanguify nitrogenous, albuminous foods. When foods adapted to stomach digestion are eaten, less nerve force is expended, for the first three hours after eating, than is required to liquefy the cereals ; and at the end of the three hours the bulk of the work has been accomplished, much of the food elements have been assimilated, and the work remaining to be done when the residue is passed on to the second stomach is comparatively insignificant. Not so the starch foods. The first three hours are consumed in an abortive effort at digestion; more vital force is consumed than is needed in digesting and assimilating those foods adapted to stomach digestion ; and, when the contents are passed on to the intestines, substantially the whole work of digestion—preparation for assimilation—yet remains to be done. And this is why those persons whom Dr. Salisbury or Mrs. Stuart are able to persuade to confine themselves to an exclusively meat supper soon find that they sleep much better, and also feel themselves very greatly improved. The vital energy is not consumed in laborious and protracted efforts to digest food which is wholly unsuited to the human stomach ; the vital force being conserved, and the nerves not tired, insomnia is overcome ; and with sleep—" Nature's sweet restorer "—there is a continual augmentation of nerve force, of vital power, and of health ; and these results are accomplished by the Salisbury treatment, not because it is a meat diet, but because it is in substitution for a food natural to cattle, but wholly unsuitable to the human stomach, and in spite of the excremental and poisonous nature of animal flesh.

In the quoted extract, Mrs. Stuart tells us that she still considers Vegetarianism the ideal diet ; but, she says, the trouble is we have not an ideal stomach with which to digest it. Here lies Dr. Salisbury's and Mrs. Stuart's mistake. It is necessary that we have foods adapted for stomach digestion, and fortunately it is not necessary to resort to animal flesh to obtain these foods. Dr. Salisbury taboos sweet fruits, because he says those foods ferment in the stomach; I freely grant that they ferment in pathological stomachs, but I am also prepared to affirm and to prove that they do not ferment in physiological stomachs ; and, moreover, the sugar in those fruits is at once taken into the circulation, and at once becomes assimilable food. It will be found also that the banana is rich in nitrogenous element, and that this element is readily acted upon by the gastric-juice. Dr. Salisbury makes the great mistake of concluding that man's anatomical structure proves him to be a meat-eating animal, whereas comparative anatomy shows that the ape family are not only the most like the human animal, but their anatomy is in many ways scarcely distinguishable from the human, and the ape in his native wilds, filled with overflowing vigour and health, lives exclusively on fruits and nuts.

Sweet fruits, although well adapted to stomach digestion, are yet not adequate ; nuts contain an important and indispensable element in man's food. It is quite true that many persons cannot eat nuts without suffering from digestive difficulty ; but what is true of sweet fruits is also true of nuts —physiological, healthy stomachs find no difficulty in their digestion and assimilation ; and it will one day be seen to be an indispensable element in our dietary. If man does not get this necessary food in that product which Nature has prepared for us, you will see him reaching after substitutes, and find him eating milk, butter, cheese, and the flesh of animals. Fortunately for Vegetarians, and all those food reformers who are glad to avoid excremental food and the sin of taking life, milk and its products, and eggs, are not excremental ; they are a secretion, and not an excretion, and may be used in substitution for nuts when these are not to be had in right varieties and condition ; but man's nature will insist on having a substitute. And this is why Sylvester Graham and the Vegetarian Society, in a half-century of earnest work, have made so little headway. "Truth is mighty, and will prevail " ; but the substitution of a food designed for cattle, and utterly unfit for a human stomach, for those foods which Nature designed for us, is not in accordance with truth, and the instinct of civilisation has cried out against it.

There remains to be considered another very important result caused by the laborious, protracted, and vital-force wasting digestion of starch and cereals. Constipation has always been recognised as destructive to the well-being of our physical condition. Dr. Abernethy, a hundred years ago, proclaimed three prime rules of health : " Keep the head cool, keep the feet warm, and keep the bowels open." When we eat such foods as are adapted to stomach digestion, the nutritive value of the food is largely assimilated while still in the stomach ; and, when the residue is passed on to the intestines, what nourishing element still remains is soon absorbed into the circulation, and the remaining portion easily and quickly discharged from the bowels. There is a force or power controlling the vital processes of our organisms, that seems instinct with life, and to work with intelligent design. When foods are taken into the system which are difficult of digestion, and when this process is delayed hours beyond what is necessary or natural, this mysterious something, that watches over our animal economy, insists first and foremost that our bodies be furnished with nutrition ; our very life depends upon it ; and if food has been taken that gives up its nutrition tardily and with difficulty, this mysterious something (Nature) insists upon retaining such food until its nutriment is absorbed ; and when this is accomplished there results lethargy, and a sluggish vitality unable to expel the residue from the body. I consider cereals and starch foods the father-and-mother of constipation.

I pray my brothers and sisters in food reform to spare themselves a resort to innuendo, sarcasm, or to personal epithets or anathema. I have but one aim—to know the Truth. Having retired from the practice of medicine, Mrs. Densmore and I have no patients to seek, no books to sell, and through patients or books or this discussion not a shilling to gain ; and I shall endeavour not to be deterred from the investigation of a Truth, however unpopular, and however severe the epithets that may be hurled at me.

# Part III.

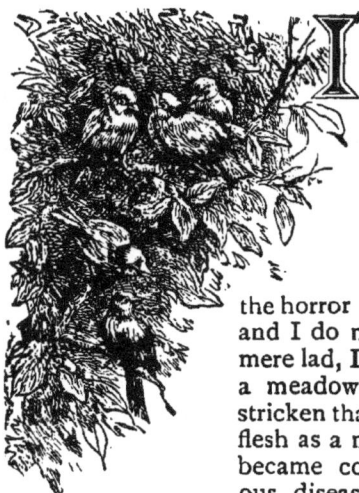

BECAME a convert to Vegetarianism from physiological rather than ethical reasons ; more from its relation to the health of man, than to the cruelty to animals. At the same time, my instincts were always in the right direction. In childhood, reared on a farm, I always sought refuge in flight when a chicken or any animal was to be killed ; I was greatly interested in fishing, but gave it up from the horror I felt upon seeing a fish torn from the hook ; and I do not recollect firing a gun but once ; when, a mere lad, I accompanied some boys hunting, I aimed at a meadow-lark, and wounded it, but was so horror-stricken that I have never lifted a gun since. But I ate flesh as a matter of course ; and gave it up only when I became convinced that it is an excremental, poison-ous, disease inducing food.

Coincident with the espousal of Vegetarianism, I became convinced that man, through transgression of natural law, and especially through errors in diet, has greatly shortened his natural term of life on earth ; that the "threescore years and ten" is a statement of the term to which he has fallen, not been designed. Naturalists teach that the number of years which animals usually live is about six times the time required for maturity ; 6 by 20 make up the 120 years mentioned in Genesis, and the term which I believe to be man's natural life-time on earth. I was (and am still) intensely interested in this subject of the longevity of man ; and in the same year that I became a Vegetarian I learned of a book enti-tled, *How to Prolong Life : an Enquiry into the Cause of Old Age and 'Natural Death' showing the Diet and Agents best Adapted for a Length-ened Prolongation of Existence,* by Chas. W. De Lacy Evans, M.R.C.S.E., Surgeon to St. Saviour's Hospital, and author of several scientific works of great interest (Baillière, Tindall, & Co., King William-street, Strand). I purchased a copy at once, and found it valuable for its extensive tables of the analysis of foods (I had a copy of the first edition, the tables have been condensed in the second), and for the numerous satisfactory and confirmatory instances of very great longevity—some of them almost rivalling the age of the patriarchs.

But at this time I regarded wheat as man's ideal food ; and I was so disgusted, on a casual glance at the contents, to find Dr. Evans pointing out cereals as the most unfavourable food for man, and stigmatising bread as the "staff of death," that I threw the book aside, refusing to read it, concluding that, however great my possible longevity, life is too short to waste on what I, with complacent bigotry, had concluded, without reading and without investigation, to be a meaningless tirade. Mrs. Densmore read it at the time, and was enough interested in Dr. Evans' views to ask me to answer several questions concerning it ; still, my precious life was too short, and I remained an entirely self-satisfied and owl-wise bigot. If my Vegetarian brethren refuse to read my recent contributions on the subject of flesh diet and cognate matters, and refuse to answer the question I have with some persistence pressed home to them, I am in no situation to complain.

Dr. Evans starts with the proposition that the ossification and deposit of earthy matter in the joints and tissues of the aged—with the resultant weakness and decrepitude—is not the result of "old age," but that old age is the result of ossification and the deposit of earthy matter in the system, and that this deposit of earthy matter is directly traceable to easily avoidable errors in diet. Dr. Evans acknowledges his indebtedness to "Patriarchal Longevity," by "Parallax," "in which," he tells us, "ossification as a cause of old age was first pointed out"; and also his indebtedness to "Records of Longevity," by Easton and Bailey, and to Hufeland's "Art of Prolonging Life," edited by Erasmus Wilson, F.R.S. The great interest attaching to this subject is my excuse for the following somewhat lengthy extracts from Dr. Evans' book :

"In every being throughout animated nature, from the most insignificant insect to the most enlightened, ennobled, and highly developed human being, we notice a deeply rooted love for one possession before all others, and that is the possession of *Life*. What will not a man give to preserve his life ? What would he not give to prolong it ? The value of riches, titles, honour, power, and worldly prospects are as nought compared with the value which every sane man, however humble, and even miserable, places on the preservation of his life. . . .

"The laws of life and of death, looked upon in this light, form the basis of a fixed science—the Macrobiotic, or the art of prolonging life. There is, however, a distinction to be made between this art and the science of medicine, but the one is auxiliary to the other.

"There is a state of body which we term *health ; plus* or *minus* divergences from this path we call *disease*. The object of medicine is to guide these variations to a given centre of bodily equilibrium ; but the object of the Macrobiotic art is, by the founding of dietetic and other rules, on general principles, to preserve the body in health, and thereby prolong life.

"In the present work the author has attempted to go beyond this, by enquiring into the *causes* which have a share in producing the changes which are observed as age advances, and, further, by pointing out a means of checking them. 'He who writes, or speaks, or meditates, without facts as landmarks to his understanding, is like a mariner cast on the wide ocean, without a compass or a rudder to his ship.' If he conceives an

Idea, a phantom of his own imagination, and attempts to make it a reality by accepting only those facts or phenomena which accord with his premature conception, ignoring those which contradict this shadow or idea, but which may nevertheless be demonstrably true, he creates a *theory*, which may be incorrect, and if so is doomed, sooner or later, to destruction. Although it possibly required but a few hours to construct, centuries may elapse before it is finally destroyed. The founder of an erroneous hypothesis creates a *monster*, which only serves to combat and stifle *Truth*. The struggle can last for a time only, for Truth must of necessity ultimately prevail. . . .

" It has long been the opinion of scientific men, that by suitable diet and regularity the blessings of life may be enjoyed in fair health to a ' green old age.' The purpose of this work is to show that we may for a time curb the *causes* which are visible in *effect* as age advances, and thus prolong life ; and, further, that by other means, founded upon simple fact, we may accomplish this for a lengthened period.

" The author's attempt to deal with a matter of such vast importance as the prolongation of life will necessarily subject him to severe and probably adverse criticism. In the first edition of a book hurriedly written in moments snatched from the turmoil of a general practice, many minor errors are sure to be found ; but, as the author takes facts for a beacon, there is no error in principle. He will only ask those who criticise to imagine themselves for the time in the position of Astræa, the goddess of Justice, and not to weigh the evidence with one scale heavily laden with prejudice. . . .

" With all our physiological, anatomical, and philosophical discoveries, there are left many questions at present not solved ; amongst others, the action of the brain, thought, motion, life, and the possible prolongation of existence. Nature speaks to us in a peculiar language, in the language of phenomena. She answers at all times questions which are put to her ; and such questions are experiments.

" In ' old age ' the body differs materially from youth in action, sensibility, function, and composition. The active, fluid, sensitive, and elastic body of youth gradually gives place to induration, rigidity, and decrepitude, which terminate in ' natural death.' In nature there are distinct reasons for every change, for development, growth, decomposition, and death. If, with our minds free from theory, and unbiassed by hypotheses, we ask Nature the cause of these changes, she will surely answer us. Let us ask her the cause of these differences between youth and old age—why the various functions of the body gradually cease ; why we become ' old ' and die. The most marked feature in old age is that a fibrinous, gelatinous, and earthy deposit has taken place in the system ; the latter being composed chiefly of phosphate and carbonate of lime, with small quantities of sulphate of lime, magnesia, and traces of other earths.

" Among physiologists and medical philosophers generally, the idea prevails that the ' ossification ' (or the gradual accumulation of earthy salts in the system) which characterises ' natural death ' is the *result* of ' old age,' but investigation shows that such an explanation is unsatisfactory. For, in the first place, if ' old age ' (which is really the number of years a person has lived) is the cause of the ossification which accompanies it, then, if ' like causes produce like effects,' *all* of the same age should be found in the same state of ossification ; but investigation proves beyond all doubt that such is not the case. How common it is to see individuals about fifty years old as aged and decrepit as others at seventy or eighty ! . . . .

" We now come to the most important change of all, which fully accounts for the many differences in the brain existing between youth and old age, that is, the changes in the blood-vessels supplying it. The arteries in old age become thickened and lessened in calibre from fibrinous, gelatinous, and earthy deposits. This is more easily detected in the larger vessels ; but all, even to the most minute subdivisions, undergo the same gradual change. Thus the supply of blood to the brain becomes less and less ; hence the diminution in size of the organ from the prime of life to old age; hence the functions of the brain become gradually impaired; the vigorous brain of middle life gradually giving place to loss of memory, confusion of ideas, inability to follow a long current of thought, notions oblivious of the past and regardless as to the future, carelessness of momentary impressions, softening of the brain, and that imbecility so characteristic of extreme age."

After quoting from Copland, Hooper's "Physician's Vade-Mecum," and from the experiments of M. Rayer, M. Cruveilheir, M. Rostan, M. Recamier, and others, Dr. Evans continues:

"We have quoted from the above authorities to show that ossification and thickening of the arteries of the brain has not been overlooked, but that it is a fact which has been known for many years; also to show that this gradual process of ossification is not due to any inflammatory action.  And we shall show that this earthy matter has been deposited from the blood, and increases year by year with old age, thus lessening the calibre of the larger vessels, partially, and in some cases fully, 'clogging up' the capillaries, gradually diminishing the supply of blood to the brain, causing its diminution in size in old age, and fully accounting for the gradual loss of the mental capabilities before enumerated.

"As age advances, the energies of the *ganglial system* decline; digestion, circulation, and the secretory functions are lessened; the *ganglia* diminish in size, become firmer, and of a deeper hue.  In old age the *nerves* become tougher and firmer, the medullary substance diminishes, and their blood-vessels lessen in calibre.  The sensibility of the whole cerebro-spinal system decreases, hence diminution of the intellectual powers, lessened activity and strength in the organs of locomotion in advanced age."

I quote further, from pages 27 and 28:

"In the foregoing pages we have pointed out the differences existing between youth and old age.  In the former the various organs and structures are elastic, yielding, and pliable; the senses are keen, the mind active.  In the latter, these qualities are usurped by hardness, rigidity, and ossification; the senses are wanting in susceptibility, the mind in memory and capacity.

"Further, that these changes are due, firstly, to a gradual accumulation of fibrinous and gelatinous substances; secondly, to a gradual deposition of earthy compounds, chiefly phosphate and carbonate of lime.  These, acting in concert, diminish the calibre of the larger arterial vessels, and by degrees partially, and sometimes fully, obliterate the capillaries.  By these depositions every organ and structure in the system is altered in density and function; the fluid, elastic, pliable, and active state of body gives place to a solid, inactive, rigid, ossified, and decrepit condition.  The whole system is 'choked up'; the curtain falls, the play of life is ended, terminating in so-called 'natural death.'

"The general impression is that this accumulation of fibrinous, gelatinous, and osseous matter is the *result* of old age—the result of time, the remote *effects* of the failure of that mysterious animal principle, life  But in an after chapter we shall show that this great vital principle, which is centred in the cerebro-spinal axis, gradually wanes because the brain and nerves by degrees lose their supply of blood, their powers of selection and imbibition, and are deprived of their ordained nourishment by means of this gradual process of induration and ossification.  . . .

"We will now enquire into the *source* of these depositions, which gradually accumulate from the first period of existence to old age.  . . .

"As the *blood* is built up from the *chyle* (which is formed from the chyme by the action of the bile and pancreatic fluid), we should expect to find in the latter the same calcareous matter ; *and such is the fact,* that, on analysis, we find the same earthy salts in the chyle as exist in the blood. As the *chyle* is formed from the *chyme* (which is the product of the action of the stomach and its secretions on food), we should in it find the same calcareous matter ; and such, again, is the *fact.* But as the *chyme* is the product of *digestion,* we expect to find the same calcareous matter in the contents of the stomach ; and such also is the *fact.* The contents of the stomach consist of food and drink taken to nourish and support the system, and in that food and drink we ought to find the same calcareous substances ; and chemical analysis gives to us the certain answer, that the food and drink taken to support the system contain, besides the elements of nutrition, *earthy salts,* which are the *cause* of ossification, obstruction, old age, and natural death.

"We have now traced these earthy compounds which are found in the system, and which increase as age advances, to the blood, from which they are, by the process of transpiration, gradually deposited. From the blood we trace them to the chyle, from the chyle to the chyme, aud from the chyme to the contents of the stomach and thence to articles of diet. Thus we eat to live, and eat to die.

"As we have traced these earthy salts to our food or articles of diet, we naturally inquire whether the different kinds of food and drink, which we have for our selection, contain the same proportion of ossifying and ' old age ' producing matter. Here chemical analysis answers in the negative ! Some of the most generally used alimentary substances contain a comparatively *large* proportion of earthy compounds, some a *moderate,* and others a very *small* amount. ' No matter what kind of food we eat, or what fluid we drink, the earthy salts contained therein have all the same source—the earth.'

" If we eat vegetable food, plants derive their earthy salts from the earth in which they grow. If animal flesh be our sustenance, they have the same source, through the medium of the animal we eat, which derives its supply from vegetation. Fish in the sea, fowl in the air, animals upon the earth, all derive the earthy salts contained in them originally from the earth, in the food on which they live. Any organ, or all the organs put together, of man or any being, cannot *generate* any element ; hence *all that is earthy in man is derived from the earth.*

" From this it follows, that if we can so regulate our diet—food and drink—that the amount of earthy matter taken into the system be sufficient only for the growth and nourishment of the bones, without which our powers of strength and motion would be useless (the body being deprived of its mechanical levers), the many organs and structures would not, and could not, harden and ossify ; the arteries would not become indurated and lessened in calibre, capillaries would not become obliterated, the brain would not decrease in size by age, sight would not fail, hearing, taste, and smell would not lose their susceptibility, hair would not turn grey, the skin would not become dry and wrinkled, the body would retain its fluidity, elasticity, and activity, and the brain its mental capabilities. If we can so regulate our diet that these earthy compounds are taken into the system in *smaller* quantities, and therefore take a *longer* period to accumulate—if we can even partially accomplish this—we can prolong life !

" We have shown ' old age ' and ' natural death ' to be due to *two* causes—*firstly,* to the action of atmospheric *oxygen,* which consumes our bodies and causes fibrinous and gelatinous accumulations ; *secondly,* to a deposition of *earthy* matter (ossification). If, therefore, we can, by artificial means, partially arrest the never-ceasing action of atmospheric oxygen, and at the same time prevent the accumulations of these earthy compounds, or even remove them from the system—that state of body termed ' old age ' would be deferred, and life would be prolonged for a *lengthened period !*

" Liebig says : ' Many of the fundamental or leading ideas of the present time appear, to him who knows not what science has already achieved, as extravagant as the notions of the alchemists.'

"In all the animal kingdom there is a beauty of structure manifested, wondrous, marvellous, and exquisite ; but man *alone* has bean endowed with knowledge, wisdom, and understanding, as a sole and exclusive gift to him.

"Speaking of the patriarchs, Josephus affirms : ' *Their food was fitter for the prolongation of life ;* and besides, God afforded them a longer time of life on account of their virtue, and the good use they made of it in astronomical and geometrical discoveries.' Many authors contend that the years, at the time of the patriarchs, were shorter than at the present time—not more than one-fourth the period. If this were true, Methusaleh would have lived only two hundred and forty-three years, Terah fifty-one, and Abram forty-four. Enoch would have been only sixteen when he begat Methusaleh, Arphaxed eight and three-quarters when he begat Salah, Salah seven years old when he begat Eber, and Adam would have been more than a great-grandfather at thirty-three. There is no evidence to show the years were less than at the present time. It is probable, and quite possible (presuming that their diet tended to longevity), that the patriarchs lived to their recorded ages. Who, therefore, can deny that, with all our knowledge and discoveries, which are daily increasing, man may not again re-discover the secret of long life, which has been lost for so many ages, and which secret may probably be summed up in the following few words :

"If a human being subsists upon food which contains a large proportion of lime, a large proportion will enter into the composition of the chyme, the chyle, and the blood ; and as from the blood the deposition of lime takes place, the greater the amount of lime that blood contains, the greater will be the amount deposited in the system, the greater the degree of ossification, and the sooner will be produced that rigidity, inactivity, and decrepitude, which make him old and bring him to *premature death.*

"On the other hand, if the food and drink taken to nourish and support the body are selected from the articles which contain the *least* amount of lime, the least amount will enter into the composition of the chyme, the chyle, and the blood, the less amount will there be to deposit, the less the degree of ossification, the less the rigidity, inactivity, and decrepitude, and the *longer the life of the man !*"

Dr. Evans gives over twenty pages to tables of the analysis of foods, which show that fruits and nuts have the least proportion of earthy matter, as compared with their nourishing properties, of any of the foods now used by man ; next in order are animal foods ; then come vegetables, third in the order ; and fourth and last are the pulses and cereals, which are shown to have the largest amount of earthy matter. The following quotation is from page 74 :

"From the foregoing analyses we see that fruits, as distinct from vegetables, have the least amount of earthy matter : most of them contain a large quantity of water, but that water in itself is of the purest kind—a distilled water of nature, and has in solution vegetable albumen.

"We also notice that they are to a great extent free from the *oxidised* albumens—glutinous and fibrinous substances, and many of them contain *acids*—citric, tartaric, malic, etc.—which, when taken into the system, act directly upon the blood, by increasing its solubility, by thinning it ; the process of circulation is more easily carried on, and the blood flows more easily in the capillaries (which become lessened in calibre as age advances) than it would if of a thicker nature. By this means the blood flows easily in vessels which have been perhaps for years lost to the passage of a thicker fluid. Further, these acids *lower* the temperature of the body, therefore the process of wasting, combustion, or oxidation, which increases in ratio to the temperature of the body, as indicated by the thermometer. . . .

"Speaking of the *ancients*, Hesiod, the Greek poet, says: 'The uncultivated fields afforded them their *fruits*, and supplied their bountiful and unenvied repast.' Porphyry, a Platonic philosopher of the third century, a man of great talent and learning, says: 'The ancient Greeks lived entirely upon the *fruits* of the earth.' Lucretius, on the same subject, says:

"'Soft acorns were their first and chiefest food,
And those red apples that adorn the wood.
The nerves that joined their limbs were firm and strong ;
Their life was healthy, and their age was long. . . .
Returning years still saw them in their prime ;
They wearied e'en the wings of measuring Time :
Nor colds, nor heats, on strong diseases wait,
And tell sad news of coming hasty fate :
Nature not yet grew weak, not yet began
To shrink into an inch the largest span.' "

I hope my readers have carefully read the preceding extracts from "How to Prolong Life." If so, it will be clearly seen that Dr. Evans has made a most valuable contribution to a vegetarianism in the absolute sense—to living on food procured exclusively from the vegetable kingdom. And since fruit is universally admitted to be the ideal and aesthetic diet, advanced Vegetarians may well rejoice over Dr. Evans' championship of an exclusively fruit diet.

In addition to those arguments in favour of fruit eating, with which Vegetarians are familiar—namely, that fruits abound in cooling and corrective acids, that they are filled with water more exquisitely distilled than science can yet compass, and that their free use opens the portals of the system and cures and prevents many diseases—Dr. Evans contends (in which view I do not concur) that the amount of needed nitrogen in food has been very much over-estimated, and that fruit eaters can get this nitrogen in some mysterious way from the atmosphere ; and he has made, in my judgment, a most important contribution to advanced Vegetarianism, in pointing out that nuts and fruits are the most free of all foods from earthy matter, and hence from liability to cause ossification and decrepitude.

Earnest attention is called to the following further extracts from Dr. Evans' book. It will be seen that he places fruits and nuts as first in their fitness for the promotion of health and longevity ; animal foods are placed second ; vegetables third ; and last, and worst, are placed the pulses and cereals, which, from their excess of earthy salts, are of all foods best calculated to induce ossification of the joints and tissues, thickening of the arteries, and consequent and inevitable premature old age, and that decrepitude and imbecility universally but wrongly reckoned a necessary condition of senility.

It is curious and interesting to observe that this order, in which Dr. Evans has classified foods, corresponds with what all philosophical students will agree must have been the experience of the race since its entry upon our planet. At first man, with no tools, agriculture, or fire, could neither kill or catch animals, raise cereals, or cook either the one or the other ;

and must have subsisted—like all animals below man—on foods spontaneously produced by nature; hence nuts and fruits must have been the first foods utilised by man. Next came the slaying, cooking, and eating of animals; wild tribes of men existing on the earth to-day are substantially unacquainted with cereals and agriculture, subsisting on foods spontaneously produced, supplemented by the flesh of animals. And last comes agriculture and cereal eating.

The consensus of writers, from the time of the Greeks to the present day, unite in saying that the primitive peoples had health and vigour; while it has been reserved for Civilisation to breed diseases whose names are legion, and to witness imbecility, decrepitude, and premature death go hand in hand with luxury and plenty. The race has strayed far from the path of health and peace; and most likely must return by the route whence it came : (1) Discontinue the use of cereals and vegetables, and the multitudinous cookings and concoctions to which the use of these products give birth; (2) Make fruits and nuts the basis of human food, supplemented by such animal products, with the minimum of cookery, as in the present condition of the race may be found necessary; (3) An absolute return to nuts and fruits, uncooked and unseasoned. After which there will be no diseases, and no doctors, upon the face of the earth.

"It *is* one of *nature's laws,* and a very simple one, that we are built up from what originally was vegetable albumen; and, with the exception of the alkaline and earthy salts, every structure and organ in our bodies was developed from and is nourished by albumen. It *was* one of the laws of Eden that man should eat albumen—vegetable albumen—in its purest form, as it exists in fruits.

"There is, therefore, a simplicity, a reason, a wonderful philosophy in the first command given to man. Man may live entirely upon fruits, in better health than the majority of mankind now enjoy. Good, sound, ripe fruits are never a cause of disease; but the vegetable acids, as we have before stated, *lower* the temperature of the body, decrease the process of combustion or oxidation—therefore the waste of the system—less sleep is required, activity is increased, fatigue or thirst hardly experienced: still the body is well nourished, and, as a comparatively small quantity of earthy salts are taken into the system, the *cause* of ' old age ' is in some degree removed, the *effect* is delayed, and life is prolonged to a period far beyond our ' threescore years and ten.'

"*Animal flesh,* taken as a class, contains, next to fruits, the least amount of earthy salts. . . .

"The amount depends, *firstly,* upon the quantity contained in the food of the animal; *secondly,* upon the duration of time the animal has eaten such food—that is, its age. Younger animals of every class contain a less amount of earthy salts in their flesh than older ones; thus veal, in the analyses generally given, contains only about one-fourth the amount of earthy salts found in an equal weight of the flesh of an adult animal, and it further contains from 12 to 15 per cent. more phosphoric acid than is necessary for the formation of salts. . . .

"' The true unsophisticated American Indians near the sources of the Missouri, during the winter months, are reported to subsist entirely upon dried buffalo flesh—not the fat portions, but the muscular part. . . . During their subsistence on dried *pemmican,* they are described by travellers, who were intimate with their habits of life, as never tasting even the most minute portions of any vegetable whatever, or partaking of any other variety of food. These facts, then, tend to show that *albuminous* tissue is of *itself* capable of sustaining life.'—*Dr. Thompson.*

"In other articles of animal food we have *milk*, unskimmed, skimmed, and butter-milk; they all contain about ·7 per cent. of salts; but the latter contains a large quantity of lactic acid, which has a great tendency to prevent the accumulation of earthy matter in the system.

"*Cheese* contains salts in about the same proportion as milk deprived of its water. It seems by its analysis to have a large quantity of salts (nearly 5 per cent.), but they exist in ratio to its highly nourishing properties.

"Eggs contain 1·5 per cent. of salts (·5 per cent. less than beef and mutton). . .

"The cereals constitute the basis of man's food; they mostly contain large quantities of mineral matter, and as a class are the worst adapted as a food for man, in regard to a long life. Man's so-called 'staff of life' is, to a great extent, the cause of his premature death.

"In the twenty-second and twenty-third chapters of the Third Book ('Thalia') of Herodotus, describing a visit of some Persian Ambassadors to the long-lived Ethiopians (Macrobii), the Ethiopians 'asked what the Persian King was wont to eat, and to what age the longest-lived of the Persians had been known to attain. They told him that the King ate *bread*, and described the nature of *wheat*—adding that *eighty years* was the longest term of man's life among the Persians. Hereat he remarked, "It did not surprise him, if they fed on *dirt* (bread), that they died so soon; indeed, he was sure they never would have lived so long as eighty years except for the refreshment they got from that drink (meaning the wine), wherein he confessed the Persians surpassed the Ethiopians." The Ichthyophagi then, in their turn, questioned the King concerning the term of life and diet of his people, and were told that most of them lived to be *a hundred and twenty years old*, while some even went beyond that age: they ate *boiled flesh*, and had for their drink nothing but *milk*.' . . . .

"We, therefore, see that the different kinds of food, in regard to longevity, have the following order: fruits, fish, animal food (flesh, eggs, etc.), vegetables, cereals. In the same order do we trace the age of man by his diet. It is written that man in the first ages lived for a period which to us seems incredible; but in the present generation the average time of life is so short, that a man at eighty or ninety years is truly a modern 'patriarch.' Man's first and ordained diet was fruits; he then ate animal food, which was subsequently permitted to him; after this he gained a knowledge of agriculture—he grew vegetables and cereals; and, not content with this, during the last few years he has learned to add lime artificially to them—to shrink and lessen an already shortened existence.

"In nature a curious yet simple phenomenon is often observed—a *rise* and *fall*. If perpetual, it alternates and becomes a fall and rise. We notice it in the sun, in gravity, in fluctuation, in the tides, and even in the rise and fall of empires. Man has degenerated —this degeneration is due solely to his diet. He has *fallen*; but we hope that he has *risen* to the highest point in the art of shortening his days, and that in the present generation he will commence to gradually *fall* back on his original and ordained diet. Since the creation, the days of man's existence have been little by little decreasing—it has been a gradual *fall*; but both science and religion tell us that he must *rise* again, that his life on earth must be prolonged. . . . .

"It is a well-known fact that children brought up on *human* milk are healthier and more robust than children fed on cow's milk. The reason is obvious. The salts in *human milk* exist in ratio to its nourishing properties, as one part of salts to seventeen and a half parts of nitrogenous matter; in *cow's* milk, as one part of salts to six and one-third parts of the same nourishing substances. Therefore, in round numbers, the nutrient part of cow's milk contains nearly three times the amount of salts as compared with human milk. The proportions of alkaline and earthy salts are proximately the same in the ashes of both, so that one ounce of caseine taken from cow's milk contains nearly three times the amount of *earthy* salts found in an equal weight of caseine from human milk.

"A human being takes four or five times longer to mature than a cow; the latter therefore grows more quickly, and its bones ossify in a less period of time than the former, whose organs are more gradual in their development and growth—whose bones should take a longer time to ossify, and therefore nature gives a food which contains less *earthy* matter. If we do not follow nature's laws, some bad result must follow, and one-half of our strumous children, who, besides their milk, are as a rule fed on bread and other farinaceous foods—most of them rich in earthy compounds—are for their age, in years and months, bodily older than healthy and robust children of the same age. Rickets and mollities ossium are in themselves diseases, not necessarily caused by a deficiency of earthy salts in the food, but by a lack in the system of power to assimilate them.

"We can stunt the growth of the lower animals by giving them an excess of earthy matter; we can ossify them, make them permanently old, and shorten their days, by the same. In human beings we need not look further than the Cretins found in the valleys of the Alps, Pyrenees, and other regions. Although cretinism has two distinct causes, the first and most important is that an excess of *earthy* matter—lime or magnesian lime—is taken into the system in solution in water used for drinking purposes. Hereditary it must be to children born of parents suffering from this disease, if not removed from the cause; but sound healthy children brought into districts where cretinism exists are, at an early age, equally subject to the disease with children born in them.

"Now these beings are, in their infancy, literally prematurely ossified, the development of the bones is arrested, the height being seldom more than four and a half feet. The bones of the cranium, which in a natural state should expand to allow the brain to grow and develop, at an early age become thickened, hardened, and ossified to such an extent that expansion is impossible; the brain, therefore, cannot develop; it is gradually deprived of its blood-supply from below; it is encased and imprisoned by its own shield; its intellectual part cannot develop; the being is subservient to the animal portion; he becomes voracious and lascivious, and in many cases sinks in intelligence below the level of many of the brutes. The age of Cretins is short; few of them reach thirty years, and, as Clayton remarks, 'although they die early, they soon present the appearance of age.' This miserable state of existence is due, to a great extent, to *premature* ossification. . . . .

"As we know there are many who could not be persuaded to make any alteration in the *articles* of their diet, whilst there are others who might be influenced in this direction, we give a few rules for both these classes. To those who are not inclined to alter the articles of their diet, we say :

"1. Eat *moderately*, always remembering that you eat to live—to give a balance to the system.

"2. Take no more than three meals a day.

"3. *Avoid* eating *large quantities* of bread, pastry, and other farinaceous foods.

"To those who are willing to make alterations in their diet, the same rules will apply, but with this difference : Eat *fruits*, if possible at every meal, and commence with them ; if the appetite is not moderately satisfied, finish with the ordinary articles of diet."

I have heard it said that a prominent Vegetarian, in a public address, recently stated that if he could be persuaded that he could live twenty years longer by going back to a meat diet, he would not think of making the change ; "because," said he, "a Vegetarian life is so much more jolly, and one enjoys life so much more while one does live." I am reminded that this is almost the exact reply that is quite universally made to me by the flesh-eater, when pleading with him to adopt the more clean and more wholesome diet of the fruit-eater. And the answer, in both cases, is made in entire ignorance of the law of life. Lest any one attempt to be " jolly " by a liberal indulgence in champagne, or tobacco, or any of the so-called pleasures of life ; and afterwards let the same person adopt only water or fruit for drink, and wholly abstain from all poisons ; and he will find that any one who seeks pleasure in poisons makes a great mistake— that the life of the water drinker is productive of far more pleasure, and is far jollier, than is possible to the wine drinker.

At the same time, it is now quite well known—thanks to the Temperance reform—that indulgence in spirit tends to shorten life, and abstemiousness tends to longevity. This will be found to be a universal law, that whatever mode of life tends to promote health and vigour, tends also to promote the " jolliest " life, and the happiest, and at the same time conduces to a prolonged life ; that whosoever foregoes twenty years, that his briefer life may be jolly, loses at every point—he always curtails his usefulness, as well as minimises his enjoyment of life ; and that whosoever adopts a course of living that promotes longevity will find himself brimful of useful energy, and usefulness is the secret of a really jolly life.

Lack of space forbids more than a brief quotation from Dr. Evans' chapter on " Instances of Longevity in Man and in the Animal and Vegetable Kingdoms." I quote from page 99, and following pages :

"On reviewing nearly two thousand reported cases of persons who lived more than a century, we generally find some peculiarity of diet or habits to account for their alleged longevity ; we find some were living amongst all the luxuries life could afford, others in the most abject poverty, begging their bread ; some were samples of symmetry and physique, others cripples ; some drank large quantities of water, others little ; some were total abstainers from alcoholic drinks, others drunkards ; some smoked tobacco, others did not ; some lived entirely on vegetables, others to a great extent on animal foods ; some led active lives, others sedentary ; some worked with their brain, others with their hands ; some ate only one meal a day, others four or five ; some few ate large quantities of food, others a small amount ; in fact, we notice great divergence both in habits and diet, but, in those cases where we have been able to obtain a reliable account of the diet, we find one *great cause* which accounts for the majority of cases of longevity, *moderation in the quantity of food.* . . .

" Charles Macklin, of James'-street, Covent Garden, an eminent dramatic writer, and comedian of Covent Garden Theatre, the veteran father of the stage, died in 1797, aged 107. In the former part of his life he lived intemperately ; subsequent thereto, he determined to proceed by rule, which he scrupulously observed.

" ' *He was moderate at his meals,* and ate fish, flesh, etc., till the age of seventy ; when, finding tea did not agree with him, he substituted milk, with a little bread boiled in it, sweetened with brown sugar. . . . For the last forty years, his principal beverage was white wine and water, pretty sweet. . . . He strictly observed the dictates of nature, ate when hungry, drank when thirsty, and slept when sleepy.'—*Vide* Memoirs of his life. . . . .

" ' Margaret Robertson, or Duncan, the oldest woman in Scotland, died at Coupar Angus yesterday. She was born in 1773, and her husband, a weaver, died fifty years ago, and left her with a daughter, who is still alive, and over sixty. Mrs. Duncan was a *heavy smoker*, and until recently, when she became blind, was in possession of all her faculties. Her last illness was only of a week's duration.'—*Daily Telegraph*, September 17, 1879.

" We do not advise either drinking or smoking, as a means of prolonging life ; but still there is a philosophy noticed in the cases before us. Both drinking and smoking take away the appetite ; less food is eaten, therefore a less amount of earthy salts are taken into the system, and the cause of old age is delayed in its results ; still sufficient food is taken to support life, and great age follows. . . .

" Among other instances of longevity we have the ancient Britons, whom Plutarch states ' only *began to grow old* at 120 years.'

" ' They were remarkable for their fine athletic form, for the great strength of their body, and for being swift of foot. They excelled in running, wrestling, climbing, and all kinds of bodily exercise ; they were patient of pain, toil, and suffering of various kinds ; were accustomed to fatigue, to bear hunger, cold, and all manner of hardships. They could run into morasses up to their necks, and live there for days without eating.'— *Henry.*

" Boadicea, Queen of the ancient Britons, in a speech to her army, when about to engage the degenerate Romans, said : ' The great advantage we have over them is, that they cannot, like us, bear hunger, thirst, heat, or cold ; they must have fine bread, wine, and warm houses ; to us every herb and root are food, every juice is our oil, and every stream of water our wine.'

" ' Their arms, legs, and thighs were always left naked, and for the most part were painted blue. *Their food consisted almost exclusively of acorns, berries, and water.'*— *Goldsmith.*

" From the above, we may justly infer that the ancient Britons lived on a diet which contained comparatively a small amount of earthy salts ; further, the acorn contains tanno-gallate of potash, which would harden the albuminous and gelatinous structures : they would therefore be less liable to waste and decay. Their endurance of hunger, cold, and hardships, and their love of water (probably from a hardened state of the skin), cannot be considered as mere fables. . . . .

" Thomas Parr, a native of Shropshire, died in 1635, aged 152. He married at the age of eighty-eight, ' seeming no older than many at forty.' He was brought to London by Thomas, then Earl of Arundel, to see Charles I., ' when he fed high, drank plentifully of wines, by which his body was *overcharged*, his lungs obstructed, and the habit of the whole body quite disordered ; in consequence, there could not but be speedy dissolution. If he had not changed his diet, he might have lived many years longer.'— *Easton.*

" On his body being opened by Dr. Harvey, it was found to be in a most perfect state. ' The heart was thick, fibrous, and fat ; *his cartilages were not even ossified, as is the case in all old people*,' and the only cause to which death could be attributed was a ' mere plethora, brought on by more luxurious living in London than he had been accustomed to in his native country, where his food was plain and homely.' In a poem by John Taylor, on ' the old, old, very old man,' the following outline of his diet is given :

> " ' He was of old Pythagoras' opinion,
> That green cheese was most wholesome with an *onion*
> Coarse meslin bread, and for his daily swig,
> Milk, *buttermilk*, and water, *whey*, and whig.
> Sometimes metheglin, and for fortune happy,
> He sometimes supped a cup of ale most nappy.'

" He was married a second time at the age of a hundred and twenty-one, and could run in foot-races and perform the ordinary work of an agricultural labourer when a hundred and forty-five years old. . . .

" Miguel Solis, of Bogota, San Salvador, who is supposed to be at least one hundred and eighty. At a congress of physicans, held at Bogota, Dr. Louis Hernandez read a report of his visit to this locally famous man, a country publican and farmer.

" ' We are told that he only confesses to this age (one hundred and eighty years) ; but his neighbours, who must be better able to judge, affirm that he is considerably older than he says. He is a half-breed, named Miguel Solis, and his existence is testified to by Dr. Hernandez, who was assured that, when one of the " oldest inhabitants " was a child, this man was recognised as a centenarian. His signature, in 1712, is said to have been discovered among those of persons who assisted in the construction of a certain convent (Franciscan convent, at San Sebastian). Dr. Hernandez found this wonderful individual working in his garden. His skin was like parchment, his hair as white as snow, and covering his head like a turban. He attributed his long life to his careful habits ; *eating only once a day*, for half an hour, because he believed that more food than could be eaten in half an hour could not be digested in twenty-four hours. He had been accustomed to *fast* on the first and fifteenth of every month, drinking, on those days, as *much water* as possible. He chose the most nourishing foods, and took all things cold.'—*Lancet*, Sept. 7th, 1878.

" From this and other sources we gather the following habits of this man : (1) He eats but once a day, and only for half an hour. (2) He eats meat but twice a month ; from which we may justly infer that he is to a certain extent abstemious in his daily meal. (3) He drinks large quantities of water. (4) He fasts two whole days every month.

"From these habits it follows that, compared with the majority of mankind, he eats little, yet enough to support life ; he therefore takes into his system a small amount of earthy compounds, which therefore take a longer period to accumulate, and produce the symptoms of decrepitude and old age at a far later period than they occur in most individuals who live upon an ordinary quantity of food, whose bodies become rigid, decrepit, and ossified, we will say, at about 'three-score years and ten.' Further, that his drinking large quantities of water, which, if not unusually hard, will tend to dissolve and remove those earthy compounds, which are not the *effect* but the *cause* of old age. We have not thought it necessary to make further inquiries concerning the diet and habits of this man. Our information is derived from numerous periodicals, and we only arrive at the above conclusions because we are convinced, from ascertained facts and experiments, that man may by diet alone attain the age which Miguel Solis is supposed to be."

My concluding quotations from Dr. Evans' erudite, logical, and remarkable book begin on page 176 :

" Science dictates, and even the most casual observer who—for purpose or principle—attempts to comprehend the truths and phenomena of universal Nature, unhesitatingly admits, that 'every *phenomenon* has its *reason*, every *effect* its *cause*.' This is a fact established and indisputable ; but how often are the *laws of life* and *of death* doomed to be overlooked by the deluded, and even removed from their legitimate situation, which they of necessity embrace in forming volumes in the library of the academy of Nature ! For the sake of method, we classify and arrange under many heads, which are but servitors to avoid a chaos of observations, descriptions and deductions ; the confusions thus avoided obviously present themselves, but one branch of science is dependent upon another—each forms a part, all united a whole—for Nature is one. To recognise one and ignore another portion or an entirety—each part of which is dependent upon unity—is to break a rule which remains unbroken. To say that everything dies simply because it has lived —that the age of man is *fixed* irrespective of reason or cause—is not only presumption, but confessedly a want of conception, a disbelief in what is and therefore must be, and an assault on the fixed and immutable laws of natural phenomena.

" When we reflect or meditate on the progress of civilised man, we notice wonders and improvements in his surroundings, for his welfare and comfort; we discover a spirit of enquiry amongst men, a silent march of thought—a steady progress, impelled forward by an eternal law—Nature's law—experience. This law we may compare to a circle; the beginning we know not, the end we know not. This circle enlarges, expands—where is the limit? Opposition, reproach, threats and violence can only be a temporary check; they cannot control, abate, or arrest the progress of enquiry, the keenness of research, the results of experience. But amongst the varied and expanding objects of research, is not enquiry which appertains to the preservation of life the most important of all to humanity?

" What is man without health, even if endowed with riches? Take away the latter and their accompanying luxuries—only give him health; this accomplished, the first desire is a return of the riches. But with both a word remains which we hate to utter, a thought we dread to contemplate, a thing which gives sorrow, pain and grief. That word, that thought, that thing, is *Death*. Even in cases where life appears a burden, how tenaciously do men cling to it! How the spirit recoils from a struggle with Death! How fondly it retains its grasp of life! Man's great desire is for health and long life on earth; to this there are but some few exceptions—the result of incidental impressions. ' Man clings to the world as his home, and would fain live here for ever.'

" ' And can we see the newly-turned earth of so many graves, hear the almost hourly sounding knell that announces the departure of another soul from its bodily fabric, meet our associates clad in the garb of woe, hear of death after death among those whom we knew—perhaps respected, perhaps loved—without pausing to consider if we may not seek and haply find *more than the mere causes*, find the *means of checking* the premature dissolution that so painfully excites the deepest and most hidden sympathies of our nature? *The prolongation of the life* of the people must become an essential part of family, municipal, and national policy. Although it is right and glorious to incur risks and to sacrifice life for public objects, it has always been felt that length of days is the measure, and that the completion by the people of the full term of natural existence is the groundwork of their felicity. For untimely death is a great evil. What is so bitter as a premature death of a wife, a child, a father? What dashes to the earth so many hopes, breaks so many auspicious enterprises, as the unnatural death? The poets, as faithful interpreters of our aspirations, have always sung, that *in the happier ages of the world this source of tears shall be dried up.'—Registrar-General of England.*

" In the present day, when we are so accustomed to wonders that they no longer excite our wonder; when we send our thoughts almost round the world with the velocity of lightning; when we hear voices miles away by the agency of the telephone; the tick of a watch—even the tramp of a fly—by the microphone; when we transcribe the vibrations of sound with the precision of a mathematician; when we freeze water into ice in white hot crucibles; when we cast copper into statues without the aid of heat; when it is possible to illuminate cities without gas—with lamps devoid of flame or fire; when some of the most precious minerals are produced from their elements; when we believe that to-morrow even the diamond may be artificially produced; with all these wonders recently brought to light for the benefit of mankind, is man *himself* to be debarred from that social progress which is daily manifested? Are the achievements of science of no avail in benefiting his degenerated existence? Will not our daily increasing knowledge of Nature and the behaviour of her elements eventually tend to this end? In reference to which Liebig asks : ' Is that knowledge not the *philosopher's stone*, which promises to disclose to us the laws of life, and which *must finally yield to us the means of curing diseases and of prolonging life?'*

"The fields of research become richer and wider with every new discovery, which is often as precious, if not more useful, than gold—actually a transmutation for the benefit and comfort of man. But as yet he has *himself* been little benefited by science, which must of necessity ultimately dictate a *means* of curing diseases and of prolonging life. Is it even just, in the present day of so-called wisdom, to ridicule the alchemists of old, who diligently laboured and searched for a 'virgin earth'—a mysterious substance which would 'change the baser metals to gold, and be a means of curing diseases, of restoring youth to the exhausted frame of age, and of prolonging life indefinitely'? Such a view would be utterly unjust. For the present science of chemistry owes its position, its existence—perhaps its origin—to the untiring observations and researches of the alchemists, which were instilled into them in their laborious searches for the 'philosopher's stone.' All they sought for exists, and may ultimately be found in the illimitable science of chemistry. . . . .

"The beneficial effects of fruit as an article of diet, both in health and disease, cannot be overrated. In health, the apple, the pear, the grape, the strawberry, the gooseberry the tomato, the fig, the date, wall-fruits, the melon, and numerous others, present such a field for choice that the most capricious appetite need never be disappointed. The supply of fruit in the United Kingdom is not great, but considerable quantities of both fresh and preserved fruits are imported from all parts of the world, and are rapidly becoming popular amongst all classes ; and it is to be hoped that our fellow-countrymen will gradually become more alive to the benefits to be derived from a more general and frequent use of fruits as an article of daily food.

"'When pain and anguish wring the brow,' in slight and temporary indisposition, or during prolonged febrile diseases, what is more refreshing and beneficial than the juice of the luscious orange ? Indeed, in many parts of the world, especially in tropical regions, the juice of the orange taken in large quantities has been found to be a specific for many descriptions of fever ; it is, in fact, Nature's remedy, and an unsurpassed one.

"Cereal and farinaceous foods form the basis of the diet of so-called 'Vegetarians,' who are not guided by any *direct* principle, except that they believe it is wrong to eat animal food. For this reason Vegetarians enjoy no better health, and live no longer, than those around them. Our remarks, therefore, apply to fruits as distinct from vegetables. . . . .

"In conclusion, we may say that, although the desire for long life exists as a natural, prevalent, and deeply-rooted love, there are, through continued trial and disappointment, many exceptions : in fact, the present subject is not acceptable to all. Our remarks are therefore confined to those who believe that, 'In this world there is, or might be, more sunshine than rain, more joy than sorrow, more love than hate, more smiles than tears. The good heart, the tender feeling, and the pleasant disposition make smiles, love, and sunshine everywhere.'"

To my mind, the unfitness of cereals, pulses, and starchy vegetables as food for man, is proven by the diseases (diabetes and obesity) that are directly traceable to these foods, and which are usually cured (or, at least, greatly mitigated) by the elimination of these foods ; and this conclusion is greatly strengthened and confirmed by the well-known fact in physiology, that starch foods are not adapted to stomach digestion, and can only be prepared for assimilation in the more protracted and nerve-force exhausting digestion in the intestines. This discovery, or illumination, came to me, so far as I know, quite independently of the labours or researches of other workers in the field of food reform. The reader will readily appreciate my delight, upon first reading Dr. Evans' book, to find further proofs and confirmations of the unsuitable nature of cereals as food. I was greatly delighted, not only to find my views confirmed and re-affirmed, but from an entirely different standpoint. Truth is homogeneous ; its parts are always related, and agree. I feel grateful to Dr. Evans for his able and convincing proof that cereals and pulses are, of all accustomed foods, most inimical to man.

At the same time, I must utter a word of caution to readers of this valuable book. Dr. Evans is not emancipated from the superstition of drug medication. Iron is a necessary constituent of the blood, and old-school practitioners have the delusioh that they can nourish with inorganic iron ; whereas it has been plainly proven that only the iron which has been organised in plant growth can be assimilated—that which is administered in medicine is wholly excreted, and the stimulation following its administration is the result of irritation. Dr. Evans likewise makes the mistake of recommending phosphoric acid, the product of a series of retorts and involved distillations, seemingly unacquainted with the plain fact that Nature's laboratory yields a product of a far more exquisite nature than man-made chemistry even borders upon ; and not knowing that man can best get all his needed acids, and phosphorus, and all else, from the fruits of the earth. Moreover, Dr. Evans plainly inculcates the doctrine that tea and coffee are valuable as foods, and that a moderate use of tobacco is desirable for those who can endure it ! Dr. Evans also makes the mistake of supposing that, since the race have used cereals for generations, generations will be required before we can safely wholly do away with these foods, whereas I have myself abstained practically—not only from bread, but all cereals and vegetables—for nine months, and have made more marked improvements in my health in that time than before during an eight years' experience in Vegetarianism.

In my next, I will offer some deductions drawn from the theory of Vital Food, and from the higher aspects of Vegetarianism, favouring nuts and fruits as the natural food of man, and excluding cereals, pulses, and vegetables.

# Part IV.

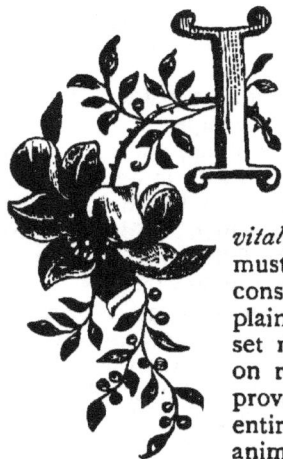

I DO not deem myself competent, at this writing to express an opinion as to the correctness or incorrectness of Mr. Hills' theory of Vital Food; I have not given the subject adequate consideration. In regard to the bearing of some of the necessary postulates of that theory, I desire to call the attention of my readers.

It will be seen at a glance that a food, to be *vital*, in accordance with the theory of Vital Food, must be taken uncooked and unseasoned. Let us consider, first, the matter of rawness. It must be plain to the philosopher and scientist that at the outset man—without fire or tools—must have subsisted on raw food. That this food was fairly adequate, is proven by the fact that the race exists; that it was entirely adequate, is probable from the fact that all animals below man, living upon raw foods, and foods spontaneously produced by Nature, are in the most robust, vigorous health; and there is no reason why man should be an exception to the rule. Tried by this test, what do we find? Fruits and nuts are exquisitely adapted to our needs and desires, in a state of nature. But how fare other foods? Science teaches that all starch foods are made more nutritious and digestible by cooking, since the sac containing the starch granule is softened and opened by the process, and the adapted digestive juices, coming in contact with the nutriment contained in the starch granule, proceed at once to the work of preparing it for assimilation and nourishment. If cereals are eaten raw, a large proportion of the starch granules pass through the digestive tract unopened, and have no other effect upon the organism than the wasting of the vital force required in the process of eliminating these (in such condition) valueless products from the system. The universal instinct and custom of cooking cereals—in all climes, and in all ages—is in accordance with the teaching of science in this matter, and it will be found that a custom coextensive with the race always has a basis for its existence other than custom.

This law, that cooking improves the digestibility of cereals, is not confined to the human animal. In America, where large numbers of cattle are fattened for the markets, it is customary to feed raw maize to the cattle ; the excrement from these cattle is then given to swine, which seem to fatten as readily on the excrement as the cattle on the raw maize (usually called corn in America); and thousands of swine are thus annually fattened, whose only food is the excrement from maize-fed cattle. Within a stone's-throw from the publication office of the *Vegetarian* is exposed for sale a large cooking-vat, or boiler, in which English farmers improve their starch foods for their cattle. It has been seen, from a preceding chapter, that starch foods at their best are not adapted to stomach digestion, and necessarily require a protracted and vital-force wasting process ; but, from the higher aspects of Vital Food, it will be seen that, if we are not permitted to cook our cereals, still more are we obliged to discard them from our dietary. As for raw pulse, the very thought is repulsive to the last degree ; the most enthusiastic devotee of Vital Food will hardly be stout-hearted enough to make the attempt of eating raw pulse undisguised and unmixed with a less repulsive food ; and are our tastes and instincts to stand for nothing ? Raw wheat, decorticated, is not repulsive ; but, with the bran unbroken, it will be found a food too difficult of mastication for the human grinder, and, even when thoroughly masticated, there remains a large amount of indigestible bran, which food reformers in America have shown to be productive of inflammation of the stomach and intestines.

When Mr. Hills tells us that " there are many foods of the muscles and many foods of the mind, many foods of the soul and many foods of the spirit," I feel like asking for some evidence of these assertions, drawn from the teachings of science, or deduced from the facts of human experience ; and I feel very sure that, if a score of men and women—Vegetarians or not, believers in Vital Food or not—are given a plentiful supply of raw foods, consisting of the best varieties of fruits, nuts, cereals, and pulses, and are not permitted to have any other food, it will soon be seen that they partake most of fruits, somewhat liberally of nuts, next to none of cereals, and absolutely none of pulses.

It will be seen that the facts of seasoning tell as conclusively in favour of a diet of nuts and fruit, and against a diet of cereals and pulses, as the matter of non-cooking. From my adoption of Vegetarianism, some eight years since, I was intuitively convinced that all animal products, and all salt and seasonings, are wrong. I tried for years to abstain both from salt and animal products. I found, after a two years' trial, that I could get on very well on a diet of fruits and cereals unsalted, with the addition of milk ; and also found that I got on nicely on a diet of fruits and cereals, without any animal products, with the addition of salt. I was as full of theories as need be ; and theoretically I was opposed to both animal products and salt ; practically, I was forced to use the one or the other. These facts had been a puzzle to me for years ; when, reading, in the *Vegetarian Messenger* for March, 1890, a review of Dr. Holbrook's book, entitled "Eating for Strength," light began to dawn. The following somewhat lengthy quotation from this review clearly points out a scientific reason why salt is necessary where cereals, pulses, and vegetables form a considerable portion of man's diet.

" Let us now look at the potash and soda salts. Potash is a very remarkable material ; phosphate of potash is an essential constituent of the muscles, and also of the blood corpuscles. In the serum of the blood, however, it is an abnormal constituent, causing paralysis of the heart and frequently sudden death. One may, without especial danger, take chlorate or carbonate of potash through the stomach, as is often the case by prescriptions of physicians. The same dose, or even a less one, however, introduced directly into the circulation, causes death. . . "Johannus Ranke says that potash is a substance which, if it accumulates in the flesh cells or nerve cells, causes irritation of the muscles and paralysis of the nerves. We find here a riddle. How is it that this material is a necessary constituent of the firm material of our bodies, but so deadly in the serum of our blood ? Dr. Bunge suggests that the potash and soda salts decompose each other, as is the case when mixed in the laboratory and allowed to crystalise, new compounds being formed, one being chloride of potassium and the other carbonate of soda.

" Another fact comes to light in this investigation, that the plant-eating animals require more common salt than the flesh-eating ones. Some of them are so greedy for salt that they will travel long distances to salt-licks in order to obtain it, which is never the case with carnivorous animals. Now, if we compare the food of the flesh-eaters with that of the herbivora, we find about the same amount of chloride of sodium (common salt), but the amount of potash salts in the food of vegetable-eating animals is from two to four times as great. Bunge suggests that the reason why the vegetable-eaters require more salt is to decompose or change the form of the great excess of potash salts, which we have seen may be very injurious ; or may not the potash draw so heavily on the chloride of sodium in the body as to make the addition of it in our food necessary in order to maintain the equilibrium of the body ? In order to test this question scientifically, Bunge made an experiment on himself. First, he ate food for five days with such exactness as to bring the excretion of the salts to a regular and constant amount. On the fifth day he added to his food eighteen grammes of phosphate of potash. Although he had not added any chloride of sodium, there was not only an immediate increase of excretion of potash salts, but of soda salts also. Repeated experiments gave the same results. He estimated that, by the addition of twelve grammes of potash salts to the food, nearly half of the soda salts of the blood would be extracted. This, he thinks, proved his hypothesis. Potash in small quantities withdraws from the body chloride and sodium, or its oxide, soda, both constituents of common salt, and this requires the addition of it to our food.

" It may be seen at a glance that all vegetables contain less soda than milk ; and they all contain, rice excepted, more potash than this article. If potash, as shown by Bunge, withdraws soda from the body, it may be seen that the addition of common salt to the food poor in soda is a scientific necessity.

"We also see why a babe nourished on its mother's milk does not require the addition of common salt. Its food contains less potash salts and more soda salts than almost any other article of food.

" Liebig remarked that there seemed to be a popular instinct to add more salt to those articles of food which were rich in starch, as, for instance, wheat-meal, peas and beans, and it seems that these are the very ones which contain most potash.

"In this connection it may be remarked that potash salts in large quantities affect unfavourably the mucous membrane of the digestive tract, and especially the stomach. Consequently, all those who suffer from weakness of the stomach should avoid potatoes, and substitute rice instead.  Rice is also more easily digested than potatoes for other reasons.  It contains less cellular or woody and indigestible matter enclosing the starch cells. One writer on food (Mulder) goes so far in his opposition to potatoes as an article of diet as to declare it would be a blessing to the race to banish them from the planet and substitute rice.

"Dr. Bunge has collected facts concerning the use of salt among various people.  He finds that those who live mainly on flesh, as hunters, fishermen, and nomadic tribes, do not care for salt.  Of the Samoyden he says :  'They know nothing of bread, and but little of roots.  Flesh and fish constitute their daily food.  The use of salt is unknown, though easily attainable from the sea.  The Tungusen eat no raw flesh, but cook it in fresh water and use no salt on it.  The Dolganen and Juralkan, in North Siberia, possess many salt nines, but they never use salt, unless as a medicine.  Their food is fish and reindeer flesh.'  Wrange writes concerning the Tschuktschen :  'Their food is flesh, and they use no salt, but have actual repugnance to it.'

"Prof. Schwartz dwelt in the land of the Tungusen three years ; lived on the flesh of wild birds and reindeer without the addition of salt, and felt no need for it.

"There are tribes of flesh-eating men in both tropical India and Africa who use no salt ; they even laugh at those who do use it.

"On the other hand, most of the native tribes of Africa cultivate the soil.  Mungo Park says :  'The Mandigos breakfast early on porridge made of meal and water, flavoured with the rind of tamarind to give it relish.  About two they eat a meal consisting of pudding made of corn meal, milk, and vegetable butter.  Their chief meal is eaten late at night, and consists of broth made with corn-meal, wheat-meal with vegetables, with sometimes a little flesh and vegetable butter.  They are principally Vegetarians.'  Concerning salt, he says :  'They have a great craving for it.  If a child gets a piece of rock-salt from a European, it eats it as our children do sugar.  The poorer classes look upon a man who can afford salt as a rich man.'  Park's own experience was that he had a painful craving for salt, which could not be described.  On the west coast of Africa a man would sell his wife or child for salt.  A war for a salt-spring between different tribes is not uncommon. To them salt is no luxury, but a necessity.   .  .  .

"Many of the facts and statements of this chapter are drawn from German sources, and especially from a little work entitled, 'Die Modernen Principien der Ernahrung,' nach v. Pettenkofer und Voit, von Dr. Aug. Guckerston, a most valuable little work, putting in popular language the scientific experiments of the most learned German students of man's food—a subject now attracting more attention than at any former time."

We have in this a direct and conclusive proof that salt is needed in a diet of cereals and pulses ; ergo, if salt is an unnatural and injurious substance, cereals, pulses, and vegetables do not form any portion of the natural food of man.

There are those among us who proudly announce themselves Vegetarians from the ethical side of this question, who speak slightingly of health considerations, designating these as selfishness, and defining Humaneness to be sympathy for the sufferings of animals.  I am of a different opinion ; to my mind, the reduction of the sufferings of animals is well, is humane— the reduction of the sufferings of human beings is better, is humaner. Further, I am of opinion that lack of health and premature death are productive of far more misery on the earth than all other causes combined, and whoever does most to lead the race back to health, longevity, and consequent usefulness, wins the grand prize—becomes the first apostle of humaneness.

It is my firm resolve to plead with Vegetarians to open their eyes to the plain fact, that the results of Vegetarian propaganda are a comparative failure ; compared to its importance, it has made no progress. There must be a cause for this ; let us all join hands in an effort to discover it. My suggestion and claim, that cereals and pulses are the great stumbling-block —the scorpion which we have been hugging as it stings—demands an earnest investigation of the foundation and reasonings on which this claim is based, rather than a resort to personalities and invective. If it shall be proven, as I believe, that the starch foods are the *bête-noir* of Vegetarianism, as well as of the race, and if the abandonment of these foods leads the race back to health, then Vegetarianism—opposition to taking the life of animals—will make rapid progress, and there will be ushered in a reign of real humaneness, to man and animals alike.

If readers of the *Vegetarian* will carefully read the quotations I have made from Dr. Evans' "How to Prolong Life," and also the remarks I have made thereon, and will then carefully read Mr. Hills' criticism in the *Vegetarian* of June 28th, page 409, I am quite content to rest my case.

(1) It will be remembered that the reason why I discard cereals from my dietary is not primarily from fear of earthy deposits, as has been before pointed out ; it is because many serious and sometimes malignant diseases are directly traceable to starch foods, as is shown by the fact that these diseases are uniformly either cured or greatly modified by abstaining from these foods.

(2) The fact that the exclusion of starch foods explains the phenomena of striking cures from a meat diet, is another argument in favour of the exclusion of cereals.

(3) The success of the "grape cure," "whey cure," and "milk cure" establishments is accounted for when it is noted that these establishments exclude all starch foods, and administer those adapted to stomach digestion.

(4) It is admitted by all scientists that the cereals are a man-developed product, the result of civilisation. Primal man, having no cereals or vegetables to resort to, must have depended for food upon those nuts and fruits spontaneously produced by nature ; and these foods are substantially free from starch. The development of cereals and starch vegetables, on the one hand, and the diseases of civilisation on the other, point to the one as the cause of the other.

(5) The long-armed ape is the animal most like man, offering a striking resemblance in many ways, its skeleton and teeth being scarcely distinguishable from that of man ; this animal lives on nuts and fruits, and not on any product having any similarity to the cereals.

(6) A still stronger argument is found in the fact that the albumenoid element in nuts, the grape sugar in fruits, and the chief nutritive elements in eggs, milk, and cheese, are adapted to stomach digestion ; whilst the cereals abound in starch, which cannot be digested in the stomach, but must await the protracted and laborious process of intestinal digestion.

(7) The most convincing, important, and overwhelming argument is found in the fact that all persons at all out of health have only to try the exclusion of cereals from their dietary, to find immediate, continuous, and permanent improvement in health.

(8) It is quite true that Dr. Evans makes, as I think, a clear demonstration that cereals are most apt of all foods to induce earthy deposits in the system, and thereby cause ossification of the joints and tissues, arterial obstruction, inadequate nutrition of the brain and the entire system, and the resultant decrepitude and premature death. Many readers have received the impression that the tendency of cereals to make earthy deposits is the strongest argument against their use.

The seven reasons stated above had entirely converted my mind to the conviction that cereals must be excluded from human food, as the first and most important step towards overcoming the diseases of modern life, before I had any conviction whatever as to the importance of this eighth or Dr. Evans' reason mentioned above. I was and am much pleased with this additional and confirmatory reason, proving that cereals must be excluded from human food before health and longevity can be obtained ; but the argument most apt to make headway, in my opinion, lies in the fact that nearly all persons are out of health, and if they will substitute fruit, with eggs, milk, and cheese, for starch foods, they are quite sure to reap signal benefits ; whereas the ossification that Dr. Evans has pointed out does not usually take place until after middle life, and so many years are required to make a practical proof that human nature is apt to tire of the effort.

Mr. Hills writes : " I am profoundly convinced that Dr. Densmore is making a most lamentable mistake ; with the best of motives, he is introducing most dangerous doctrines." There has never been a new truth offered that did not, at the outset, receive this kind of opposition. I am unable to sympathise with this state of mind. The agitation of thought is the beginning of wisdom ; this is the only path to progress. The outlook, from the point of view of these " dangerous doctrines," is very different. For every Vegetarian in England, there are two to be found who have been Vegetarians, but who have felt constrained to give it up. The London Vegetarian Society, chiefly through the untiring and self-sacrificing efforts of Mr. Hills, has now for some years made herculean efforts in propaganda ; money has flowed like water, and many enthusiastic workers and speakers have been untiring in their efforts. With what results ? A number of converts to Vegetarianism are made in each winter's campaign, an equal number fall away before the year is out. Vegetarians are more confined to starch foods than they were before conversion, and are after backsliding. This is so apparent, that a correspondent in the *Times* some years since suggested that Vegetarianism ought to be called Cerealism. This greater use of the cereals has counterbalanced the benefits derived from other sources.

It is my belief that the substitution of fruit for bread and starch foods will remove from Vegetarianism its great stumbling-block ; and then the converts made in a winter's campaign will in time become centres of propaganda ; Vegetarianism "will grow on what it feeds on," all its devotees will take heart and rejoice ; the gospel of clean living, health, and humanity will overspread the earth, which shall blossom as the rose ; and every man (and woman) will literally sit under his own vine and fig-tree, partaking of their god-given fruits, and rejoicing in a life freed from pain and decrepitude, and filled with overflowing happiness and usefulness.

And the anti-cereal food crusade is not confined to Vegetarianism. Thousands who have no ear for food reform, but who are suffering from illness, will be induced to exclude cereals and vegetables from their diet; they will receive such benefits, that they will see that the food question is of great importance, and, through the influence ot these "dangerous doctrines," will be led to abstain from flesh of all kinds; this, in turn, will lessen the killing and suffering ot animals, and thus will make the heart of every Vegetarian to rejoice, whether he be a devotee of the god of Health or of Mercy.

## COMPARATIVE ANATOMY.

The Anatomical differences between flesh-eating and fruit-eating animals:—

| The Carnivora. | The Anthropoid Ape. | Man. | The Omnivora. |
|---|---|---|---|
| Zonary Placenta. | Discoidal placenta. | Discoidal placenta. | Non-deciduate placenta. |
| Four-footed. | Two hands and two feet. | Two hands and two feet. | Four-footed. |
| Have claws. | Flat nails. | Flat nails. | Have hoofs. |
| Go on all fours. | Walks upright. | Walks upright. | Go on all fours. |
| Have tails. | Without tails. | Without tails. | Have tails. |
| Eyes look sideways. | Eyes look forward. | Eyes look forward. | Eyes look sideways. |
| Skin without pores. | Millions of pores. | Millions of pores. | Skin with pores. |
| Slightly developed incisor teeth. | Well-developed incisor teeth. | Well-developed incisor teeth. | Very well-developed incisor teeth. |
| Pointed molar teeth. | Blunt molar teeth. | Blunt molar teeth. | Molar teeth in folds. |
| Dental formula: *5to8.1.6.1.5to8. 5to8.1.6.1.5to8. | Dental formula: 5.1.4.1.5. 5.1.4.1.5. | Dental formula: 5.1.4.1.5. 5.1.4.1.5. | Dental formula: 8.1.2to3.1.8. 8.1.2to3.1.8. |
| Small salivary glands. | Well-developed salivary glands. | Well-developed salivary glands. | Well-developed salivary glands. |
| Acid reaction of saliva and urine. | Alkaline reaction saliva and urine. | Alkaline reaction and urine. | Saliva and urine acid. |
| Rasping tongue. | Smooth tongue. | Smooth tongue. | Smooth tongue. |
| Teats on abdomen. | Mammary glands on breast. | Mammary glands on breast. | Teats on abdomen. |
| Stomach simple and roundish. | Stomach with duodenum (as second stomach). | Stomach with duodenum (as second stomach). | Stomach simple and roundish, large cul-de-sac. |
| Intestinal canal 3 times length of the body. | Intestinal canal 12 times length of the body. | Intestinal canal 12 times length of the body. | Intestinal canal 10 times length of the body. |
| Colon smooth. | Colon Convoluted. | Colon convoluted. | Intestinal canal smooth and convoluted. |
| Lives on flesh. | Lives on fruit. | *Homo sapiens vegetus*— Lives on fruit. | Live on flesh, carrion, and plants. |

\* In this formula the figures in the centre represent the number of incisors; upon each side are the canines, followed to the right and left by the molars.

" Man is neither carnivorous nor herbivorous. He has neither the teeth of the cud-chewers, nor their four stomachs, nor their intestines. If we consider these organs in man, we must conclude him to be by nature and origin, frugivorous, as is the ape."

www.ingramcontent.com/pod-product-compliance
Lightning Source LLC
Chambersburg PA
CBHW021520090426

42739CB00007B/699